IMPLEMENTING
CHANGE WITH
CLINICAL AUDIT

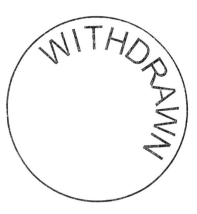

D1344894

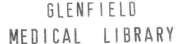

IMPLEMENTING CHANGE WITH CLINICAL AUDIT

Edited by

Richard Baker

Hilary Hearnshaw

and

Noelle Robertson
Eli Lilly National Clinical Audit Centre,
Department of General Practice and Primary Health Care,
University of Leicester, UK

JOHN WILEY & SONS

Chichester • New York • Weinheim • Brisbane • Singapore • Toronto

Other Wiley Editorial Offices 37695

John Wiley & Sons, Inc., 605 Third Avenue,
New York, NY 10158-0012, USA

WILEY-VCH Verlag GmbH, Pappelallee 3,
D-69469 Weinheim, Germany

Jacaranda Wiley Ltd, 33 Park Road, Milton,
Queensland 4064, Australia

John Wiley & Sons (Asia) Pte Ltd, 2 Clementi Loop #02-01,
Jin Xing Distripark, Singapore 129809

John Wiley & Sons (Canada) Ltd, 22 Worcester Road,
Rexdale, Ontario M9W 1L1, Canada

W
84.1
IMP

Library of Congress Cataloging-in-Publication Data

Implementing change with clinical audit / edited by R. Baker, H.
    Hearnshaw, and N. Robertson.
        p.   cm.
    Includes bibliographical references and index.
    ISBN 0-471-98257-1 (paper)
    1. Medical audit.   I. Baker, Richard H., M.D.   II. Hearnshaw, H.
(Hilary)   III. Robertson, N. (Noelle)
    [DNLM: 1. Medical Audit—methods.   2. Organizational Innovation.
3. Delivery of Health Care.   W 84.1 I34 1999]
RA399.A1I47   1999
362.1'068—DC21
DNLM/DLC
for Library of Congress   98–35855
                                                                        CIP

British Library Cataloguing in Publication Data

A catalogue record for this book is available from the British Library

ISBN 0-471-98257-1

Typeset in 10/12pt Palatino from the author's disks by Keyword Typesetting Services Ltd.
Printed and bound in Great Britain by Biddles Ltd, Guildford and King's Lynn.
This book is printed on acid-free paper responsibly manufactured from sustainable forestry, in which at least two trees are planted for each one used for paper production.

CONTENTS

Contributors   vii

Foreword   *Charles D. Shaw*   ix

Preface   xi

Acknowledgements   xv

Chapter 1   The role of clinical audit in changing performance   1
            Richard Baker

Chapter 2   Evidence and audit   21
            Richard Baker

Chapter 3   A systematic approach to managing change   37
            Noelle Robertson

Chapter 4   Overcoming obstacles to changes   57
            Hilary Hearnshaw and Richard Baker

Chapter 5   Audit and learning   69
            George Brown, Gifford Batstone and Mary Edwards

Chapter 6   Audit across interfaces   95
            M.P. Eccles, M. Deverill, E. McColl, J. Newton
            and J. Verrill

Chapter 7   Good clinical audit requires teamwork   119
            Celia McCrea

Chapter 8   Implementing change with audit: the role of
            management   133
            Jonathan Shapiro

Chapter 9   Internal communications and the management
            of change   145
            Owen Hargie and Dennis Tourish

Chapter 10   Getting the message across – language,
             translation, marketing and selling   167
             Rosalind Eve and Paul Hodgkin

      Index   179

CONTRIBUTORS

Richard Baker, Director, Eli Lilly National Clinical Audit Centre, Department of General Practice and Primary Health Care, University of Leicester, Leicester General Hospital, Gwendolen Road, Leicester LE5 4PW

Gifford Batstone, Centre for Postgraduate Medical Education, Queen's Medical Centre, University of Nottingham, Nottingham NG7 2UH

George Brown, Centre for Postgraduate Medical Education, Queen's Medical Centre, University of Nottingham, Nottingham NG7 2UH

Mark Deverill, School of Health and Related Research, University of Sheffield, 30 Regents Court, Sheffield S1 4DA

Martin Eccles, Centre for Health Services Research, University of Newcastle, 21 Claremont Place, Newcastle upon Tyne NE2 4AA

Mary Edwards, Director of Nursing and Patient Services, North Hampshire Hospitals NHS Trust, North Hampshire Hospital, Aldermaston Road, Basingstoke RG24 9NA

Rosalind Eve, School of Health and Related Research, University of Sheffield, 30 Regents Court, Sheffield S1 4DA

Owen Hargie, School of Behavioural and Communication Sciences, University of Ulster, Jordanstown BT37 0QB, Northern Ireland

Hilary Hearnshaw, Eli Lilly National Clinical Audit Centre, Department of General Practice and Primary Health Care, University of Leicester, Leicester General Hospital, Gwendolen Road, Leicester LE5 4PW

Paul Hodgkin, Institute of General Practice and Primary Care, Community Sciences, University of Sheffield, Northern General Hospital, Herries Road, Sheffield S5 7AU

Elaine McColl, Centre for Health Services Research, University of Newcastle, 21 Claremont Place, Newcastle upon Tyne NE2 4AA

Celia McCrea, Centre for Applied Psychology, University of Leicester, University Road, Leicester LE1 7RH

John Newton, Division of Employment Studies, School of Social, Political and Economic Sciences, University of Northumbria, Northumberland Building, Newcastle upon Tyne NE1 8ST

Noelle Robertson, Department of Medical Psychology, University of Leicester, Leicester General Hospital, Gwendolen Road, Leicester LE5 4PW

Jonathan Shapiro, Health Services Management Centre, University of Birmingham, Park House, 40 Edgbaston Park Road, Birmingham B15 2RT

Dennis Tourish, School of Behavioural and Communication Sciences, University of Ulster, Jordanstown BT37 0QB, Northern Ireland

Jo Verrill, Co. Durham TEC, Valley Street North, Darlington DA1 1TJ

FOREWORD

Change is the measure of audit. And audit remains central in the new world of clinical governance, as well as in the culture of professional self-regulation.

What is changing is the increasing demand from the public, patients and managers for transparent and effective mechanisms for defining, measuring and improving standards in health care. In the past 10 years in the United Kingdom there has been much attention to defining (evidence, guidelines, charters) and to measuring (indicators, audits, surveys, enquiries) but relatively little to making things happen and to closing the loop.

Even the audit enthusiasts who once argued for professional audit within a walled garden now recognize the need to involve patients, managers and the world outside. Ten years ago, professional bodies would seek to implement clinical guidelines by merely sending them to members; now they send them to purchasers and to patients. And there is a wider acceptance that clinical improvement depends more on systems than on individuals.

But we still find the technical challenges of meta-analysis and metrication more scientifically satisfying than the behavioural challenges of changing individuals and organizations. And that is the importance of this book: it is about the consummation of audit.

And, more than that, it is relevant to many other quality improvement activities which succeed only if they induce change – like confidential enquiries, accreditation, risk management. The vital ingredient is people.

Charles D. Shaw
CASPE Research
King's Fund
11–13 Cavendish Square
London W1M 0AN

PREFACE

In the past 10 years, quality improvement activities have been introduced into the health care systems of most developed countries. In the National Health Service (NHS) in the UK, clinical audit has taken a central role, but in common with other methods of quality improvement, change in performance has not always occurred. The most important part of the audit cycle is making change, but this is also the most difficult part. This book aims to provide information and suggestions about how to make change more likely.

Audit has developed from a focus on measurement to a focus on improvement. This requires identifying and implementing best practice, in turn requiring changing clinical practice or behaviour. The process of changing clinical behaviour has received more and more attention from researchers of many disciplines, from managers and policy makers. From this growing body of knowledge, we have assembled information about approaches to implementing change arising from a range of disciplines all relevant to clinical audit, and set them alongside experiences of those who have undertaken clinical audit.

We aim to encourage a systematic but practical approach, and we hope the book will be useful to all who use clinical audit, or help others in using clinical audit. In particular, we are writing for those who find the change process difficult to initiate or maintain. Health service managers who want to understand the processes involved in clinical audit may find this book helpful in identifying where difficulties may lie, and that it offers some guidance on how those difficulties might be prevented or overcome. We also hope that by bringing together information about the current level of knowledge of methods of implementing change, researchers with an interest in this field will be encouraged to explore new and possibly more promising approaches.

The book falls into two principal sections. In the first four chapters we introduce a systematic approach for implementing change in audit, and in the following six chapters other authors introduce other ideas and address particular issues in greater depth. Chapter 1 outlines the methods of audit and considers research evidence about implementing change. Although there is a choice of methods, no method is reliably effective, and it is wise to draw on a variety rather than rely on any single one. In Chapter 2, we argue that successful change depends on obtaining good quality research evidence about appropriate care, and good quality evidence about current performance.

Chapter 3 describes the concept of obstacles and levers for change, and describes a framework for identifying the obstacles and selecting particular strategies for overcoming them. This approach is based on behavioural theories about individuals, groups, and organizations, and explains why the effectiveness of implementation strategies varies when they are used in different settings and different circumstances. In Chapter 4, we show how these ideas may be used in audit in a simple and practical way. It is not necessary to be an expert in human behaviour to implement change.

Having described an approach to implementing change, invited contributors then go on to consider some of the issues in more depth, and include complementary ways to match obstacles with strategies for overcoming them. In Chapter 5, George Brown and colleagues explore the similarities between audit and learning. Evidence about learning in general, either in relation to individuals or groups, can suggest ways to make audit more effective.

Health care usually requires the collaboration of professionals from different disciplines. The challenge of collaboration can present obstacles to change, and in Chapter 6, Martin Eccles and colleagues discuss their studies of multidisciplinary audit across the interface between primary and secondary care. They relate their findings to general theories about small groups. In Chapter 7, Celia McCrea draws on evidence about groups to show how the behaviour of groups or teams involved in audit may be improved.

In Chapter 8, Jonathan Shapiro introduces the organizational factors that may influence the likelihood that change will occur. He describes how the relationship between managers and audit has evolved, and considers how a multiskilled clinical manager might emerge to integrate general and clinical management, and create culture change. The quality of communications in organizations such as hospitals or trusts can influence the effectiveness of attempts to implement change, and in Chapter 9, Owen Hargie and Dennis Tourish explore how this occurs. They suggest that investigation, and if necessary, improvement of communications should be undertaken by health service organizations to support the ability of the people in the organization to implement change. Finally, in Chapter 10, Rosalind Eve and Paul Hodgkin describe the practical use of marketing techniques. They analysed their 'market' in order to tailor the details of their methods to the needs of the health professionals with whom they worked.

By including contributors with different perspectives, we hope to show that the implementation of change in audit is subject to many influences. Factors at the organizational level include patterns of communication, and divisions between managers and health professionals, between doctors and nurses, or between primary, secondary and community care. At the level of the group or team, the effectiveness of teamwork can have a major impact on implementation, and individuals themselves may also hold attitudes or beliefs that affect the likelihood of change. If full advantage is to be taken of the opportunity that audit presents to improve the quality of care, collaboration between all levels of the health care system will be needed. Leadership from the top of the organization, open and effective communication, the reduction of fear of failure, and the support of teamwork will be needed as much as research evidence about appropriate care and the feedback of evidence about actual performance.

Richard Baker
Hilary Hearnshaw
Noelle Robertson

ACKNOWLEDGEMENTS

We would like to acknowledge the assistance of Helen Foster, Vicki Cluley and Joanna Carter, who willingly typed a succession of drafts. We also thank the editors of *Quality in Health Care* and *Audit Trends* for their permission to include material in Chapter 6 and to reproduce Figure 3.1 and Tables 3.1–3.3.

Chapter 1

THE ROLE OF CLINICAL AUDIT IN CHANGING PERFORMANCE

Richard Baker

Change is not made without inconvenience, even from worse to better – Samuel Johnson

Clinical audit is frequently used by health professionals to help them improve the quality of care. However, it is often difficult to bring about genuine changes in performance. In this chapter, we define and describe audit, discuss evidence about the strategies that may be used in audit to implement change, and identify a problem underlying most attempts to change performance – the difficulty of choosing an implementation strategy that stands a good chance of being effective.

1.1 DEFINING CLINICAL AUDIT

Audit is a term that has been applied to an enormous range of activities and in consequence many health care staff remain confused about its purpose and methods. The Concise Oxford Dictionary defines audit as an official examination of accounts. It also notes the existence of an audit ale, which was a beer of special quality formerly brewed in English colleges for drinking on the day when the audit was undertaken. Presumably the aim was to intoxicate the auditors to such an extent that they would fail to recognize discrepancies in the accounts.

An early definition of audit in health care was *the evaluation of medical care in retrospect through analysis of clinical records*, and its purpose was described as *to make certain that the full benefits of medical knowledge are being applied effectively to the needs of patients* (Lembcke, 1956). When audit was introduced into the health service in the UK, it was envisaged that it would encompass more than merely the collection of data from records. It was defined as *the systematic critical analysis of the quality of medical care, including the procedures used for diagnosis*

Implementing Change With Clinical Audit. Edited by Richard Baker, Hilary Hearnshaw and Noelle Robertson.
© 1999 John Wiley & Sons, Ltd.

and treatment, the use of resources and the resulting outcome and quality of life for the patient (Secretaries of State, 1989).

Another definition, which we prefer, highlights both the need for a systematic approach, its importance as a professional activity, and the aim of improving performance: *Audit is the process of critically and systematically assessing our own professional activities with a commitment to improving performance and, ultimately, the quality and/or cost effectiveness of patient care* (Fraser, 1982).

In many countries health care quality assurance systems have been introduced which employ a wide variety of methods including accreditation, outcome monitoring, patient surveys and financial incentives. Audit may be viewed as one form of quality assurance, but the key factors which distinguish clinical audit as undertaken in the UK from quality assurance are the two principles upon which it was established. These are that audit should (a) be led by health professionals themselves and (b) be confidential to them. Each committee or group of health professionals given local responsibility for coordinating audit has been encouraged to agree strict rules of confidentiality, so that participation can be free from risk of public censure. The rules also govern the release of information to managers and health authorities, and individuals taking part in audit can be reassured that they can identify and discuss their own weaknesses without the danger of non-participants making ill-informed judgements and imposing penalties. Thus, clinical audit can be regarded as a form of quality assurance undertaken by, and for, health professionals.

1.2   A BRIEF DESCRIPTION OF AUDIT

Audit is generally depicted as a cycle, in which standards are set, data collected, changes implemented if necessary, and followed by further data collection and review of standards (Shaw, 1980). This has much in common with the quality cycle employed in quality management (Ovretveit, 1992) or quality assurance (Ellis and Whittington, 1993), reflecting that clinical audit is one form of quality assurance. However, the apparent simplicity of the cycle may imply that progression from stage to stage is direct, inevitable and free of difficulties, when in reality the process is usually more complicated.

Instead of describing audit as a cycle, we will describe it as a process which has at least five stages: the selection of a topic; the specification of desired performance in terms of criteria and standards; the collection of objective data to determine whether the standards are met; the implementation of appropriate changes to improve performance; and the collection of data for a second time to ensure the changes have improved performance. Additional steps can include further attempts to implement change, which are followed by third or subsequent data collections.

1.2.1   Selection of a topic

If large numbers of patients are involved, and the condition carries a high risk of mortality or substantial morbidity, audit would appear to be justified. For example, hypertension is common and leads to an increased risk of premature death from strokes or heart attacks. There is also good evidence that treatment which controls blood pressure will improve outcome. Nevertheless, if care for hypertensive patients is already satisfactory, audit would produce no improvements, but if there are good reasons for suspecting a problem in the delivery of care, audit can not only be justified, but may be regarded as obligatory (Baker, 1990). In fact, there is convincing evidence that care of hypertension is often inadequate (Beevers and MacGregor, 1995). A recent study in north-west England has shown that many strokes are due to inadequate treatment, with levels below 150/90 mm Hg being required for optimal stroke prevention (Du et al, 1997). The case for an audit would appear to have been made.

Having established that an audit can be justified, an additional question must be addressed, namely what is the aim of this particular audit? In general, the purpose of audit is to improve care when it is inadequate, and in our example, the aim could be stated as 'to increase the proportion of patients with hypertension whose blood pressure is controlled'.

1.2.2   Specification of desired performance

Clarity of purpose flows from a clear expression of aims into the statements that define explicitly the level of desired performance. Performance is described in terms of criteria and associated standards. Criteria are defined as *systematically developed statements that can be used to assess the appropriateness of specific health care decisions, services and outcomes* (Institute of Medicine, 1992). They make clear what is to be measured in assessing performance; for example, a criterion included in an audit of the care of patients with diabetes might be worded as shown in Box 1.1. The criterion indicates where the information is to be found, the time period during which the examination should have taken place, and the type of examination required. It is essential that the criteria are based on good quality research evidence. If they are not, improved patient outcomes are unlikely even when compliance with the criteria improves. This issue is discussed in more detail in Chapter 2.

The standard has been defined as *the percentage of events that should comply with the criterion* (Baker and Fraser, 1995). The standard and criterion together constitute the yardstick against which actual performance is assessed.

When standards are set before collecting data, they can be used as targets, which trigger action to improve performance if they are not attained

---

Box 1.1   A criterion in an audit of diabetes care

The records show that at least annually the fundi have been examined for retinopathy by either (a) photography or (b) fundoscopy through dilated pupils.

(Lawrence, 1993). The target standard can be set at different levels. There may be particular local constraints that make the attainment of high standards difficult, for example limited resources or patients who are poorly compliant. Sometimes a standard can be set just above current performance in order to serve as a stimulus to improvement. This type of standard is referred to as a stretch standard. On other occasions, the standard is set by comparison of performance with other practitioners or organizations taking part in the audit (normative standards).

1.2.3   First data collection

Although clinical records provide the most common source of data for audit, there are many alternatives. However, the same basic principles apply whatever approach is taken. It is essential that the data are objective and accurately describe performance. The first step is to compile a complete list of patients. Second, if a sample is selected from this list, procedures must be followed to ensure that it is representative. Third, in extracting information, standard rules should be followed in order that data extractors interpret details in the same way.

The data are analysed to determine the standard of care achieved. When all relevant patients have been included rather than a sample, the findings indicate true performance. However, when samples are used, a degree of error is inevitably introduced. Provided the sample was representative, the calculation of confidence intervals can be used to take this element of error into account when drawing conclusions, the confidence intervals indicating the range of values within which the true level of performance will probably lie (see Chapter 2).

1.2.4   Implementation of change

By this point, audit has made clear why changes in performance are needed – because the topic is important, there is convincing research evidence about what care is appropriate, and there is objective evidence that current care is less than satisfactory. When implementing change, it is common to devote some time to making practical plans. The practical issues may be related to four questions – *who? what? how?* and *when?*

1.2.4.1 Who?

In making plans for improving performance, those responsible for the audit cannot usually work alone. Each of the following elements of change may involve cooperation with others. The participating health professionals may contribute to the decision about what needs changing, and how those changes are to be brought about. Health service managers might be asked to re-direct available resources, or patient groups may be asked for their opinions on the practicalities of suggested changes, or on methods to inform all patients about new service arrangements.

1.2.4.2 What?

The precise change required must be clarified. There may be several reasons for poor performance and it is essential to identify which are most important. There are techniques that may be used to pinpoint the particular problem, including fishbone diagrams, the 'five whys', and Pareto charts. Fishbone diagrams, sometimes known as cause and effect or Ishikawa diagrams (Oakland, 1993), enable a group of staff to identify the possible causes of poor performance (see Figure 1.1). Brainstorming may be used to generate suggestions to be added to the fishbone diagram. Each member contributes in turn until all possible ideas have been identified. At this stage, further discussion or formal investigation may be needed to discover which are the most important causes of problems.

The 'five whys' approach is a quality management technique that may be used to structure discussion of the suggested problems. It consists simply of asking 'why?' repeatedly until the underlying cause of a problem becomes clear. Let us take as an example an audit of blood tests for liver function before routine surgery. An audit in one surgical firm of a hospital has shown that this is common practice. Why? The junior house officers request the test – why? Because they believe it needs to be checked – why? Because when they are newly in post, the house officers are told by the ward sister that it is routine policy – why? Because the ward sister believes there is an unwritten policy about the tests – why? Because 4 years ago, a patient developed jaundice after anaesthetic, and the anaesthetist suggested that pre-existing liver disease may have been a factor.

Pareto charts are a method for displaying data about the relative importance of different causes of problems (see Figure 1.2). The choice of data needed to complete a chart may be decided following an analysis undertaken using a fishbone diagram or application of the 'five whys'. In the Pareto chart, the

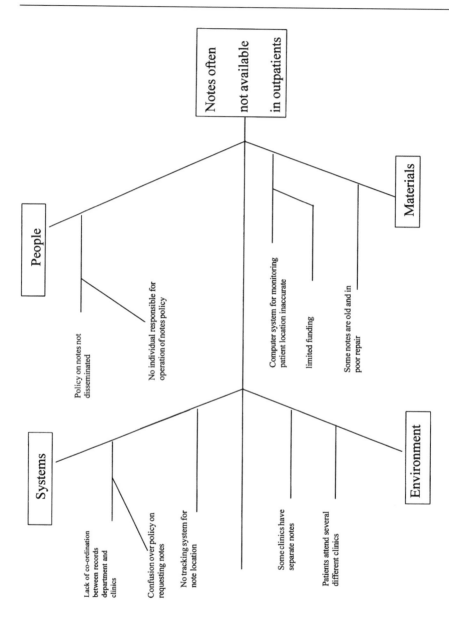

Figure 1.1 A cause and effect diagram for the problem of missing notes in outpatient clinics

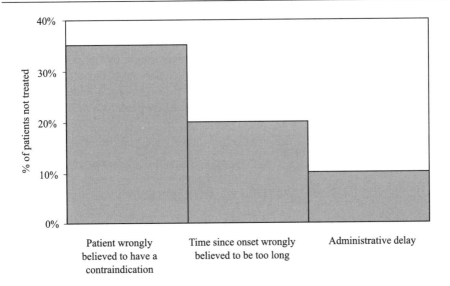

Figure 1.2 A Pareto chart of reasons for not treating patients with acute myocardial infarction with thrombolytics (patients with genuine reasons for withholding treatment excluded)

frequency with which each possible cause does actually cause a problem is displayed. This highlights which is the most important, and should be addressed first.

1.2.4.3   How?

Having decided what needs to be done by whom, a method is needed for ensuring that change does occur. It is sometimes assumed that by reaching agreement on a plan of action, those concerned will automatically change their performance. However, this assumption often proves incorrect, and additional measures are needed to implement change. In the context of professionally led, confidential clinical audit, feedback of information about performance is often the only strategy used, but many others are available. Indeed, feedback alone is one of the less effective approaches. Later in this chapter, we consider some of the alternatives.

1.2.4.4   When?

A precise timetable is required to ensure a second data collection is undertaken after the agreed changes have been given sufficient time for improvements in performance to have occurred.

1.2.5   Second data collection

Audit requires a second data collection, and this needs to be carried out as carefully as the first. The findings are compared to the criteria and standards to check that they have been achieved, and to the findings of the first data collection, to check that desired improvements have taken place.

1.3   MODELS OF AUDIT

To complete all the stages of audit described above requires motivation and effective management, particularly if relatively large numbers of professionals are involved. Various models have been used to illustrate how the stages of audit can be linked together in a managed process leading to improved performance. The most common is the audit cycle (Shaw, 1980; Lawrence, 1993), but although this describes the process, it does not fully indicate how it is to be managed. Therefore, other more complicated models have been put forward. For example, it has been argued that audit would be better represented as a spiral, with repeated data collections taking place as performance is gradually and continuously improved (Vasanthakumar and Brown, 1992).

An alternative model exemplifies the relationship between the clinical audit cycle, a change cycle, a patient care cycle and a standards setting cycle (Kogan et al, 1995). In yet another model, audit is set within a framework that ensures the health care team controls the process (Hearnshaw, 1993). Another approach envisages the audit cycle developing into the quality management cycle (Ovretveit, 1992). In this form, client and management views of quality are taken into account in addition to professionals' views, and the system has become integrated with the general management of the health care organization.

The systems adopted to manage audit and the activities of those involved in it are likely to influence its success, but evidence about the impact of such approaches on audit is limited. In this book, we will retain a distinction between audit as a five-stage process and the systems that are set up to manage it. Inevitably, such systems will be integrated to a variable extent with the general management arrangements in any particular organization.

1.4   IMPLEMENTATION STRATEGIES

In recent years, methods for implementing the findings of research and changing the performance of health professionals have been the subject of intense interest. Many good quality studies have been undertaken which provide evidence about the relative effectiveness of different methods. The findings from these studies have been synthesized in several systematic reviews.

1.4.1 Feedback

The effectiveness of feedback was addressed in an early, and unsystematic, review (Mitchell and Fowkes, 1985). Feedback was classified as either passive (supplying information about performance without any suggestions for improvement) or active (information plus some judgement about the level of performance, with or without education, guidelines or protocols). Passive feedback appeared to be relatively ineffective, but active feedback was more likely to be effective. In a more recent review of the effects of feedback (Mugford et al, 1991) 36 studies were identified, although only 11 were randomized controlled trials. Passive feedback was again found to be less effective, but active feedback was more likely to be effective, with standard setting being one strategy used to enhance the effect of feedback. In a new review from the Cochrane Effective Practice and Organisation of Care Review Group (formally the Cochrane Collaboration on Effective Professional Practice – CCEPP), audit with feedback was found to have variable impact (Thomson et al, 1997a).

1.4.2 Educational strategies

Printed educational materials are relatively ineffective. In a review of 11 studies (randomized controlled trials, interrupted time series analyses or controlled before and after studies) the effects were found to be small (Freemantle et al, 1997). The types of material included published or printed recommendations for clinical care, including guidelines and electronic publications. They could have been delivered by hand or through personal or mass mailings.

Although mailing of educational materials may have limited effect, when additional strategies are used, the chances of improvements in performance are increased. In a systematic review of the effectiveness of a variety of educational strategies in changing the performance of physicians, Davis and colleagues (1995) found 99 randomized controlled trials of strategies or interventions that objectively assessed physician performance and/or health care outcomes. The methods used to implement change evaluated in these studies included the provision of educational materials, conferences, seminars, workshops, outreach visits (see Box 1.2), opinion leaders (see Box 1.3), patient-mediated strategies (see Box 1.4), reminders (see Box 1.5) and audit with feedback. Reassuringly, 70% of the interventions demonstrated improvements in physician performance and 48% produced improvement in health care outcomes. Reminders, patient mediated interventions, outreach visits, opinion leaders and combina-

---

Box 1.2   Education outreach (academic detailing)

This marketing technique is a variant of personal selling, but is not intended to win orders for goods or services; instead the purpose is build good will. With this approach, the sales person is generally called a missionary, but in the pharmaceutical industry is also known as detailer (Zikmund and d'Amico, 1996). In adapting this method, emphasis has been placed on educating the target health professional, and therefore it has been referred to as educational outreach (Soumerai and Avon, 1990).

The outreach visit is usually brief, but meticulously planned. The objectives must be established beforehand, and characteristically some preliminary market research is undertaken to identify the issues that are likely to be important to the target professionals. It is important to establish credibility, perhaps by indicating that the detailer is a representative of a respected educational or academic organization. During the visit, the detailer explores the professional's current understanding of the topic in question and offers information required to fill the gaps in knowledge or to change opinions. Active learner involvement is sought, key messages are repeated, and simple graphical materials are left with the professional as reinforcement.

The effectiveness of educational outreach has been investigated in trials of prescribing (Avorn and Soumerai, 1983; Wayne et al, 1986; Frazier et al, 1991; Avorn et al, 1992) and appropriateness of blood transfusions (Soumerai et al, 1993). It was found to be effective in these trials, but its effect when the topics are more complex is unclear.

---

tions of methods used simultaneously were more effective, but feedback and educational materials alone were less effective. Educational conferences had relatively little impact. It should also be noted that the effectiveness of all methods varied between studies, and none could be relied upon to be always effective. The authors of this review suggested that at least part of this variation might be explained by the readiness of individual physicians to change, and noted that change appeared to occur relatively frequently in studies that addressed the barriers to change.

This conclusion is reinforced by the findings of a review of educational strategies undertaken by Oxman and colleagues (1995). They found that simple dissemination strategies such as mailed educational materials or conferences were relatively ineffective. However, more active strategies were more likely to be effective, including educational outreach, local opinion leaders, patient mediated interventions, feedback and reminders. The effectiveness of educa-

---

Box 1.3   Opinion leaders

Marketing researches have shown that the decisions are influenced by other people in the social groups to which the consumer belongs. Such groups might be clubs, associations or colleagues at work. Groups often include individuals who have particular influence because they are regarded as having expertise, intelligence or respected personal attributes (Zikmund and d'Amico, 1996). Although health professionals are taught to apply research evidence in their clinical practice, they are not immune to the influence of colleagues, and interest has grown in methods of directing this influence to control changes in performance.

The concept of social influence arises from research in the disciplines of psychology and sociology (Mittman et al, 1992). We are all liable to be influenced by what we perceive as the norms of the social environment in which we live. This influence may take place in different settings: either in one to one interactions between individuals, or in groups, or through mass media. Opinion leaders may be able to change the prevailing norms of a group of professionals, in contrast to the effect of detailing which operates at the level of the individual. The methods for using opinion leaders to change clinical practice may vary, but generally rely on providing the selected leaders with information about the research evidence and then leaving them to choose whatever approach they feel is appropriate to their setting (Lomas, 1994).

Some information is available about the effectiveness of opinion leaders in implementing changes in performance (Davis et al, 1995; Grimshaw et al, 1995). Although this does show the method can be effective, more information is needed about the selection and training of opinion leaders, their effectiveness in different settings and with different topics, and their cost-effectiveness in relation to other methods of implementing change.

---

tional outreach has recently been confirmed in another Cochrane collaboration review (Thomson et al, 1997b). Despite these encouraging findings, no single intervention was invariably effective, and in different situations, changes in care generally varied from nil to moderate.

Advice about clinical practice is increasingly being presented in the form of guidelines, which may be regarded as one variety of educational material. In a review of the implementation of clinical guidelines (Grimshaw et al, 1995), 91 high quality studies were identified, involving a wide variety of clinical settings and tasks. 87 studies examined the process of care, of which 81 reported improvements. Seventeen assessed the outcome of care, and 14 of these reported improvements. The effectiveness of different implementation strategies was variable. Educational strategies which were more likely to be effective were those that required active participation by the professionals themselves, for example targeted seminars, educational outreach visits, or the involvement of opinion leaders. Strategies were more effective if they operated during consultations between professionals and patients. These included restructured medical records, patient specific reminders during the consultation and patient mediated interventions. Despite these findings, Grimshaw and colleagues indicated that insufficient evidence was available to allow firm conclusions about the relative effectiveness of different educational and implementation strategies when used in different settings. It should also be pointed out that there has been relatively little research into methods of implementing guidelines for nurses (Cheater and Closs, 1997) or other professional groups allied to medicine.

Box 1.4   Patient mediated interventions

The use of patients to change the clinical performance of health professionals may initially appear curious. However, if the patient is provided with specific information or instructions, he or she can remind the health professional about appropriate clinical actions.

In a randomized controlled trial in UK general practice, women who received a written invitation to have a cervical smear test were more likely to eventually have a test than women who relied on being invited to have a test when they consulted their general practitioner about other problems (Pierce et al, 1989). A card carried by the patient can also be effective. In a trial of preventive health procedures such as immunization, patients who carried the card to show their physician experienced an increase in the performance of the procedures (Turner et al, 1990).

These trials suggest that patient mediated interventions are a form of reminders delivered to the professional via the patient, although originating from the health service organization. The approach appears to be suited to promoting routine procedures such as illness prevention or chronic disease management routines. Whether the method would be effective with more complex clinical procedures is uncertain. The extent to which patients could take a more active role is also unclear. Perhaps a trained and assertive patient would be able to prompt the professional even when the clinical issue is more complex.

1.4.3 Reminders

The possibility that reminders might offer one method of changing clinical performance has been suggested in several reviews discussed above. This view is supported by a meta-analysis of 16 randomized controlled trials of computer-based clinical reminder systems for preventive care (Shea et al, 1996). The trials had been undertaken in primary care settings in the USA or Canada and the findings confirmed that computer reminders were effective in improving performance of breast and colorectal cancer screening, cardiovascular risk reduction and vaccinations, but did not improve cervical cancer screening or other preventive care. A review of the impact on patient care of computers in general practice confirmed that changes in performance can occur, although the increase in the medical content of consultations may be at the expense of a reduction in patient-initiated interactions and social content (Sullivan and Mitchell, 1995).

Computers are one method of issuing reminders, but paper methods can also be employed. In a review of 20 trials of the effectiveness of strategies to increase breast screening examinations by physicians (Mandelblatt and Kanetsky, 1995), both computerized and non-computerized reminder systems were effective. Audit with feedback was also effective.

Box 1.5   Reminders

Patients may be able to remind health professionals about elements of care (see Box 1.4). Other methods can also be used to deliver reminders either during consultations or separate from consultations. Records which are structured to include prompts can act as reminders during consultations (Emslie et al, 1993). Paper reminders attached to patient records were effective in a trial of cancer screening activities by internal medicine practitioners (McPhee et al, 1989) and were also effective when used by primary care physicians (McPhee et al, 1991). However, paper reminders are not always effective (Baker et al, 1997).

Computer systems can also provide direct prompts to practitioners (MacDonald et al, 1984). Decision support systems represent a development of computer reminders. For example, a system developed in a hospital in Salt Lake City for managing antibiotic prescribing contained regularly updated guidelines in the form of rules, algorithms and predictive models (Pestonik et al, 1996). Staff were invited to pilot the system and were permitted to over rule its recommendations. Use of the system over several years was associated with increased appropriateness of prescribing and reduced cost.

1.4.4 Organizational change

The reviews discussed thus far have generally been concerned with strategies targeted directly at individuals, or relatively small groups of health professionals, most often doctors. Other types of strategy such as changes to systems of work or the restructuring of services might be equally or more effective, and may sometimes be applicable in audit, although they usually need the involvement of health service managers. However, good quality experimental studies and systematic reviews of interventions affecting the organization of services are uncommon. One review of programmes to improve primary care services was able to identify 36 studies of a variety of strategies (Yano et al, 1995). The findings suggested that different strategies were more effective for particular aspects of care. For example, successful methods for improving access to services included reorganization of professionals into teams with improved support staff and accountability, or defining and implementing specific catchment areas for all public clinics in one region. Successful methods for improving preventive activities included computer reminder systems of various types, and peer review. Specially trained nurses also improved the effectiveness of screening programmes. Effective organizational changes included assigning smaller groups of providers to a single patient receptionist, or involving at least two professional disciplines in a group or interdisciplinary team. Feedback was effective in reducing unnecessary test ordering or prescribing. However, despite the variety of strategies employed, changes to the continuity or humaneness of care and health outcomes proved difficult to implement.

Total quality management (TQM) or continuous quality improvement (CQI) is one system of organizational change. Experimental evidence about its effectiveness is limited. In a recent randomized controlled trial, CQI did not improve professionals' compliance with guidelines (Goldberg et al, 1998). The authors of this study concluded that the introduction of CQI was influenced by local organizational culture, and the people and clinical conditions involved.

1.4.5 Combinations of strategies

One approach to the problem of the variable and unpredictable effectiveness of implementation strategies might be to use combinations of strategies rather than single strategies alone. This can be compared to the clinical policy of using combinations of antibiotics to treat tuberculosis in order to overcome the possibility of bacterial resistance. In implementing change in performance, the use of combinations of strategies may be able to overcome different obstacles to change. In a review of 75 studies undertaken in primary care of combinations of strategies (Wensing and Grol, 1994), the most common combination was of feedback with either educational materials or group education. Only one-third of studies in this review were randomized controlled trials, and therefore definitive conclusions should be postponed. However, the findings do suggest that further investigation of strategy combinations is justified. The most effective combinations appeared to be individual instruction paired with a variety of other interventions, or peer review used with feedback.

1.4.6   Conclusions

The implication of these reviews is that implementing change is not simple, but neither is it impossible. In seeking to implement change, participants in audit do not need to rely on a little intuition and a lot of luck. A systematic approach is more likely to succeed, a theme to which we will return.

Despite the recent growth of research into methods of implementing change, the primary evidence and systematic reviews at present available remain incomplete. Although there are relatively more trials of strategies in primary care settings, the evidence about implementing change for every professional group is limited in both breadth and depth, and for some groups such as nurses or professions allied to medicine, there is almost no evidence at all. Some strategies have escaped detailed study. There have been relatively few trials of facilitation of health care teams, an approach that is often used in audit. Likewise, there is little controlled evidence about TQM/CQI, even though this method is sometimes strongly advocated. Advertising has received very little consideration. Furthermore, most of the trials of implementation strategies were undertaken in North America, and it is reasonable to ask whether the findings can be assumed to apply in different health care systems. Because of these limitations, firm conclusions about methods of implementing change are impossible. However, we will put forward some tentative points that might be more appropriately described as hypotheses warranting further study.

Some strategies appear to be more effective than others in particular settings and with particular topics (see Table 1.1), although it should not be forgotten that no single strategy can be relied upon to be always effective. The information contained in Table 1.1 is preliminary, and based on the limited evidence at present available about different strategies. Rather than being a definitive statement about the applicability of strategies, it should be regarded as a structure for informing the selection of strategies and stimulus for future research. However, it is clear that reliance on feedback alone cannot be justified. Those undertaking audit must draw on a wider range of appropriate strategies.

In selecting a strategy, it is important to consider the people or organizations being asked to modify their performance. The nature of the change should also be taken into account. An issue of particular importance in future research is the investigation of strategies that can be used to implement relatively complex

Table 1.1 Different strategies for implementing change, showing the targets for each strategy, the topics for which the available evidence suggests they might be applicable, and the degree to which they appear to be effective

Strategies	Target	Topic	Evidence of effectiveness
Feedback	Individuals, groups, organizations	Diverse	Variable; often less effective than other strategies when used alone
Reminders	Individuals	Circumscribed topics, e.g. preventive procedures, prescribing decisions	Relatively effective
Opinion leaders	Groups	Treatment decisions; information about impact on other topics uncertain	Variable effectiveness
Facilitation	Groups	Topics involving multi-disciplinary cooperation	Little evidence available
Patient mediated interventions	Individuals	Circumscribed topics, e.g. preventive or chronic disease management procedures	Relatively effective
Conferences	Groups	Diverse	Little or no effect
Educational materials	Individuals	Diverse	Little or no effect, unless accompanied by other strategies
Small group education	Groups	Diverse	Variable effectiveness
Educational outreach	Individuals	Circumscribed topics, e.g. prescribing decisions	Relatively effective
Total quality management	Organization	Diverse	Little information available
Reorganization of services	Organization	Diverse, including topics requiring multi-disciplinary teamwork	Relatively effective
Advertising	Individuals, groups, organizations	Unknown	Unknown

changes in performance, because much of the evidence now available relates to circumscribed aspects of performance such as prescribing decisions or preventive health checks. We have much less information about implementing change in relation to topics such as making diagnoses, professional–patient communications including explaining information about the illness and treatment options, or the management of patients when there is no clear diagnosis.

1.5 SUMMARY POINTS

- Audit is the process of reviewing the delivery of health care to identify deficiencies so that they may be remedied.
- It has five essential stages – selection of a topic, specification of desired performance, first data collection, implementation of change, second data collection.
- In planning the implementation of change, it can help to identify the prime cause of problems by applying techniques used in commercial settings.
- Feedback alone is the most common strategy chosen to implement change in audit, but there is convincing evidence that feedback alone has limited effect. Use must be made of a wider range of strategies.
- A wide range of implementation strategies is available, but although many of them can be effective, in any single audit it is difficult to predict which strategy would be the best choice.

REFERENCES

Avorn J and Soumerai SB (1983) Improving drug-therapy decisions through educational outreach: a randomized controlled trial of academically based 'detailing'. *N Engl J Med* **308**:1457–1463.

Avorn J, Soumerai SB, Everitt MD, Ross-Degnan D, Beers MH, Sherman D, Salem-Schatz R and Fields DA (1992) Randomized trial of a program to reduce the use of psychoactive drugs in nursing homes. *N Engl J Med* **327**:168–173.

Baker R (1990) Problem solving with audit in general practice. *BMJ* **300**:378–380.

Baker R and Fraser RC (1995) Development of review criteria: linking guidelines and assessment of quality. *BMJ* **311**:370–373.

Baker R, Farooqi A, Tait C and Walsh S (1997) Randomized controlled trial of reminders to enhance the impact of audit in general practice on management of patients who use benzodiazepines. *Quality in Health Care* **6**:14–18.

Beevers DG and MacGregor GA (1995) *Hypertension in Practice*. Second edition. London: Martin Dunitz Ltd.

Cheater FM and Closs SJ (1997) The effectiveness of methods of dissemination and implementation of clinical guidelines for nursing practice: a selective review. *Clinical Effectiveness in Nursing* **1**:4–15.

Davis DA, Thomson MA, Oxman AD and Haynes RB (1995) Changing physician performance. A systematic review of the effect of continuing medical education strategies. *JAMA* **274**:700–705.

Du X, Cruickshank K, McNamee Saraee M, Sourbutts J, Summers A, Roberts N, Walton E and Holmes S (1997) Case-control study of stroke and the quality of hypertension control in north west England. *BMJ* **314**:272–276.

Ellis R and Whittington D (1993) *Quality Assurance in Health Care. A Handbook*. London: Edward Arnold.

Emslie CJ, Grimshaw J and Templeton A (1993) Do clinical guidelines improve general practice management and referral of infertile couples? *BMJ* **306**:1728–1731.

Fraser RC (1982) Medical audit in general practice. *Trainee* **2**:113–115.

Frazier LM, Brown JT, Divine GW, Fleming GR, Philips NM, Siegal WC and Khayrallah MA (1991) Can physician education lower the cost of prescription drugs? *Ann Int Med* **115**:116–121.

Freemantle N, Harvey EL, Grimshaw JM, Wolf F, Oxman AD, Grilli R and Bero LA (1997) The effectiveness of printed educational materials in improving the behaviour of health care professionals and outcomes. In: Bero L, Grilli R, Grimshaw J and Oxman A (editors) Collaboration on Effective Professional Practice module of *The Cochrane Database of Systematic Reviews* (updated 2 December 1996). Available in The Cochrane Library. The Cochrane Collaboration; issue 1. Oxford: Update Software.

Goldberg HI, Wagner EH, Fihn SD, Martin DP, Horowitz CR et al (1998) A randomised controlled trial of CQI teams and academic detailing: can they alter compliance with guidelines? *Journal of Quality Improvement* **24**:130–142.

Grimshaw J, Freemantle N, Wallace S, Russell I, Hurwitz B, Watt I, Long A and Sheldon T (1995) Developing and implementing clinical practice guidelines. *Quality in Health Care* **4**:55–64.

Hearnshaw H (1993) The audit cycle managed by the primary care team. *Audit Trends* **1**:7–8.

Institute of Medicine (1992) *Guidelines for Clinical Practice. From Development to Use*. Field M and Lohr KN (editors). Washington, DC: National Academy Press.

Kogan M, Redfern S and Kober A (1995) Making audit a workable system. In: Kogan M and Redfern S (editors) *Making Use of Clinical Audit*. Buckingham: Open University Press.

Lawrence M (1993) What is medical audit? In: Lawrence M and Schofield T (editors) *Medical Audit in Primary Health Care*. Oxford: Oxford University Press.

Lembcke PA (1956) Medical auditing by scientific methods, illustrated by major female pelvic surgery. *JAMA* **162**:646–655.

Lomas J (1994) Teaching old (and not so old) docs new tricks: effective ways to implement research findings. In: Dunn EV, Norton PG, Stewart M, Tudiver F and Bass MJ (editors) *Disseminating Research/Changing Practice*. Thousand Oaks: Sage Publications.

MacDonald CJ, Hui SL, Smith DM, Tierney WM, Cohen SJ, Weinberger M and McCabe GP (1984) Reminders to physicians from an introspective computer medical record, a two-year randomized trial. *Ann Int Med* **100**:130–138.

Mandelblatt J and Kanetsky PA (1995) Effectiveness of interventions to enhance physician screening for breast cancer. *J Fam Pract* **40**:162–171.

McPhee SJ, Bird JA, Jenkins CNH and Fordham D (1989) Promoting cancer screening. A randomized controlled trial of three interventions. *Arch Int Med* **149**:1866–1872.

McPhee SJ, Bird JA, Fordham D, Rodnick JE and Osborn EH (1991) Promoting cancer prevention activities by primary care physicians. Results of a randomized controlled trial. *JAMA* **266**:538–544.

Mitchell MW and Fowkes FGR (1985) Audit reviewed: does feedback on performance change clinical behaviour? *J R Coll Phys Lond* **19**:251–254.

Mittman BS, Tonesk X and Jacobson PD (1992) Implementing clinical practice guidelines: social influence strategies and practitioner behaviour change. *Qual Rev Bull* **18**:413–422.

Mugford M, Banfield P and O'Hanlon M (1991) Effects of feedback of information on clinical practice: a review. *BMJ* **303**:398–402.

Oakland J (1993) *Total Quality Management. The Route to Improving Performance*. Second edition. Oxford: Butterworth Heinemann.

Ovretveit J (1992) *Health Service Quality. An Introduction to Quality Methods for Health Services*. Oxford: Blackwell Scientific Publications.

Oxman AD, Thomson MA, Davis DA and Haynes RD (1995) No magic bullets: a systematic review of 102 trials of inventions to improve professional practice. *Can Med Assoc J* **153**:1423–1431.

Pestonik SL, Classen DC, Evans RS and Burke JP (1996) Implementing antibiotic practice guidelines through computer-assisted decision support: clinical and financial outcomes. *Ann Int Med* **124**:884–889.

Pierce M, Lundy S, Palanisamy A, Winning S and King J (1989) Prospective randomized controlled trial of methods of call and recall for cervical cytology screening. *BMJ* **299**:160–162.

Secretaries of State for Health, Social Services, Wales, Northern Ireland and Scotland (1989) *Working for Patients* (Cmn 555). London: HMSO.

Shaw C (1980) Acceptability of audit. *BMJ* **270**:1443–1445.

Shea S, DuMouchell W and Bahamonde L (1996) A meta-analysis of 16 randomized controlled trials to evaluate computer-based clinical reminder systems for preventive care in the ambulatory setting. *J Am Med Inform Assoc* **3**:399–409.

Soumerai SB and Avorn J (1990) Principles of educational outreach ('academic detailing') to improve clinical decision making. *JAMA* **263**:549–556.

Soumerai SB, Salem-Schatz S, Avorn J, Asteria CS, Ross-Degnan D and Popovsky MA (1993) A controlled trial of educational outreach to improve blood transfusion practice. *JAMA* **270**:961–966.

Sullivan F and Mitchell E (1995) Has general practitioner computing made a difference to patient care? A systematic review of published reports. *BMJ* **311**:848–852.

Thomson MA, Oxman AD, Davis DA, Haynes RB, Freemantle N and Harvey EL (1997a). Audit and feedback to improve health professional practice and health care outcomes. In: Bero L, Grilli R, Grimshaw J and Oxman A (editors) Collaboration on Effective Professional Practice Module of *The Cochrane Database of Systematic Reviews*. Available in the Cochrane Library. The Cochrane Collaboration, Issue 1. Oxford: Update Software.

Thomson MA, Oxman AD, Davis DA, Haynes RB, Freemantle N and Harvey EL (1997b) Outreach visits to improve health professional practice and health care outcomes. In: Bero L, Grilli R, Grimshaw J and Oxman A (editors). Collaboration on Effective Professional Practice Module of *The Cochrane Database of Systematic Reviews*. Available in the Cochrane Library. The Cochrane Collaboration, Issue 4. Oxford: Update Software.

Turner RC, Waivers LE and O'Brien K (1990) The effect of patient-carried reminder cards on the performance of health maintenance measures. *Arch Int Med* **150**:645–647.

Vasanthakumar V and Brown PM (1992) Audit spiral. *Quality in Health Care* **1**:142–143.

Wayne AR, Blazer DG, Schaffner W, Federspiel CF and Fink R (1986) Reducing long-term diazepam prescribing in office practice. *JAMA* **256**:2536–2539.

Wensing M and Grol R (1994) Single and combined strategies for implementing changes in primary care: a literature review. *Int J Qual Health Care* **6**:115–132.

Yano EM, Fink A, Hirsch SH, Robbins AS and Rubenstein LV (1995). Helping practices reach primary care goals. Lessons from the literature. *Arch Int Med* **155**:1146–1159.

Zikmund WG and d'Amico M (1996) *Basic Marketing*. Minneapolis: West Publishing Company.

Chapter 2

EVIDENCE AND AUDIT

Richard Baker

When it is not necessary to change, it is necessary not to change – Lucius Cary

2.1 INTRODUCTION

Change is not always necessary. To justify change, we need convincing evidence about the appropriateness of care (research evidence), and objective evidence about our own current performance to highlight current deficiencies (performance evidence). In the absence of either of these two categories of evidence, participants in audit may reasonably ask whether they should devote time and energy to changing their performance.

Evidence about current performance may show that it is already satisfactory, and therefore change is not required. However, poor quality evidence may be worse than no evidence at all, because it may indicate that performance is satisfactory when in reality it is unacceptable. Thus, the findings should accurately distinguish care that is satisfactory from care that should be improved. If care is inadequate, the performance evidence should indicate the degree of deficiency so that the success of subsequent efforts to improve can be judged reliably.

In this chapter, we discuss the two types of evidence, both essential to implementing change. Methods of developing research evidence-based audit criteria are outlined, and the methods needed to provide objective performance evidence are described. To place these issues in context, we first consider the extent to which audit as it has been undertaken in the NHS is based on good quality research evidence about the appropriateness of care and objective performance evidence.

Implementing Change With Clinical Audit. Edited by Richard Baker, Hilary Hearnshaw and Noelle Robertson.
© 1999 John Wiley & Sons, Ltd.

2.2   A REVIEW OF PUBLISHED AUDITS

Since audit was established in the NHS, health professionals of all types, including nurses, pharmacists and therapists, have been asked to take part. It would be reasonable to ask whether all this activity has led to benefits in patient care, and to answer this question, information is needed about the quality of audits. Therefore, we have undertaken a review of published audits to identify (a) whether change took place; (b) methods of implementing change; (c) methodological weaknesses such as failure to specify research evidence-based criteria or standards, or use of methods liable to produce poor evidence about current performance. Reports of audits generally do not appear in journals that are indexed in electronic bibliographies. Therefore, we hand searched selected relevant journals (Table 2.1).

We sought papers that reported audit projects. Trials that investigated the effectiveness of audit or other methods of implementing change were excluded as these have been reviewed by others (see Chapter 1) and would be less representative of routine audits. We included only audits undertaken in the UK health service, as in other countries different systems are in place to foster quality assurance. The criteria used to judge audit methods were the five stages of audit described in Chapter 1. The findings are shown in Table 2.2.

Of the 139 audits identified that met the inclusion criteria, 61 (44%) demonstrated change by completing a second data collection to show that at least some improvements had taken place. Although the proportion of audits completing the cycle is disappointing, the level is higher than that reported in a survey of routine audits (Hearnshaw et al, 1998), perhaps because publication includes an element of selection in which those less well conducted are eliminated.

The range of methods used to implement change was relatively limited. All involved the preliminary feedback of the findings of the first data collection. Clinicians themselves, or less commonly senior nurses or clinical directors, took the lead in reviewing the findings and planning changes. The most common approach they chose was to modify systems of work, either by revising record systems or altering services in other ways, for example the introduction of a new clinic or the revision of the appointment system. Guidelines or new policies were quite common, and generally emerged from the process of discussion following feedback. No use was made of potentially more effective strategies, such as academic detailing, small group education, or opinion leaders.

In addition to the failure of the majority of the audits to demonstrate change in performance, there were many methodological weaknesses. Thirteen (21%) of the 61 audits that demonstrated change did not have explicit criteria, and instead collected data without being clear why they were needed. Of the 78 audits that did not include a second data collection, 46 (59%) did not have

Table 2.1 The journals searched to identify reports of audits (years included 1992–1996)

Audit Trends (published from 1993)
Medical Audit News (now the *Journal of Clinical Effectiveness*)
Quality in Health Care
International Journal of Quality in Health Care
Audit in General Practice (published 1993–1996)

criteria. Even when criteria were explicit, it was unusual for them to have been selected following review of research evidence. Local consensus was the most common approach. There were also many weaknesses in methods used to provide evidence about current performance, for example, it was common to find that when samples had been used, no justification for the selected sample sizes would be given. In audits using samples and with a completed second data collection, statistical tests were generally not used to check whether any observed changes could have been due to chance.

Bearing in mind that the audits in this review were selected for publication, it appears as though many clinical audits conducted thus far have major flaws in the methods used. The failure to use methods of implementing change in a systematic way is but one aspect of poor methodology in general. All too often, those taking part appear to have collected data without being clear which elements of care had been indicated by research evidence to be most important. They went on to collect poor evidence about current performance, employed methods of implementing change haphazardly if at all, and not surprisingly often gave up before collecting data for a second time.

Although few systematic evaluations have been undertaken, our review suggests that many audits have used poor methods and failed to improve care. Although many clinicians feel positive about audit, some are wary. In investigating the participation of hospital doctors in audit, Black and Thompson (1993) found that the need for audit was generally accepted, although many worries were expressed. Some junior doctors saw it as an exercise for criticizing them, and others questioned its cost-effectiveness. On the other hand, levels of participation are high among hospital doctors (Buttery et al, 1994) and general practitioners (Baker et al, 1995a). General practitioners are relatively well disposed towards audit, but face particular difficulties such as lack of time or other resources, or lack of colleagues in their primary health care teams with whom they can work (Baker et al, 1995b).

However, some clinicians have recognized that many audits fail to implement change and have suggested changes to the audit programme (see Box 2.1). In reviewing these problems, a leading medical authority on audit (Hopkins, 1996) identified a variety of problems. At the policy level, there has been confusion

Table 2.2   Findings of the review of audit reports published in journals. In some audits, more than one method of implementing change was used

Number of reports identified	174
Number subsequently excluded	
(these were not described by the authors as audit)	35
Total number of audits included	139
Number demonstrating change	61 (44%)
Methods of implementing change	
1. feedback and discussion only	17
2. development of protocols, guidelines or policies	19
3. revised record systems	8
4. organizational changes, e.g. new clinics, changed	
appointment systems etc.	20
5. other	2
total	66

between the use of audit as an educational tool for health professionals and its use for monitoring contract performance. At a practical level, there has been a long list of methodological problems. Among the solutions recommended by Hopkins was the use of methods commonplace in epidemiological studies.

Given all these methodological weaknesses and frequent failures to improve care, it is not surprising that health professionals may doubt the value of audit as it is now undertaken. However, improvement in the quality of health care will not be possible unless there is an acceptable and effective method to enable professionals to review their own performance and change it when appropriate. Thus, the routine use of audit must be improved.

2.3   EVIDENCE ABOUT APPROPRIATE CARE

In audit, appropriate care is described in terms of criteria (see Box 1.1). Criteria have been developed and used for almost as long as attempts have been made to systematically improve the quality of care. Methods for the development of criteria emerged from the movement to accredit US hospitals in the early 1950s.

Box 2.1   Disillusion with audit. Quoted from Fulton RA (1996) Audit: the emperor's new clothes. *Journal of Evaluation in Clinical Practice* **2**:199–201

Audit will never have the intellectual glamour of original research, and the need to re-audit only adds to the tedium. No amount of jargon will conceal this from busy clinicians. Doctors therefore feel bored rather than threatened by the prospect of audit, and that is why they avoid getting involved.

An important study from this period was reported by a public health physician (Lembcke, 1956). He used the case of major female pelvic operations such as hysterectomy, and assessed the appropriateness of operations undertaken by two groups of surgeons. He fed back to one group information about their performance. In this group, there was a substantial increase in the proportion of operations judged appropriate, but there was no such improvement in the control group. Lembcke recommended that criteria should be stated with precision so that they would be interpreted in the same way by different individuals, and that they should conform with generally accepted standards of good quality as described in textbooks or research studies.

2.3.1   Implicit and explicit criteria

There are two main types of criteria (see Box 2.2). In using implicit criteria, the person assessing care is usually an experienced clinician, who may have been asked to assess the care of patients whose care has been identified as possibly deficient through a preliminary screening process. This approach has been used in the context of peer review in north America, although is less common in the UK.

Because implicit criteria rely on the judgement of the assessor, the findings may not be objective, and different assessors might come to different judgements. Furthermore, because the judgements rely on opinion, they may not reflect the best available research evidence. Despite these disadvantages, there are limited occasions when the use of implicit criteria might be reasonable. For example, in risk management programmes, the care of patients who experience a marker event such as a blood transfusion reaction or a readmission might be assessed for deficiencies. Nevertheless, in audit explicit criteria should be used, and we will not consider the implicit variety further.

The early methods for developing criteria relied on the consensus opinions of panels of health professionals chosen because of their expertise or ability to

---

Box 2.2   Implicit and explicit criteria

Implicit criteria

Based on the clinical judgement of the health professional assessing care, derived during the course of the assessment

Explicit criteria

Statements agreed and recorded before the audit begins

represent their colleagues. Developments of this approach have included the assignment of different weights by the panel to different criteria, and formal processes for helping the panel reach agreement, such as the nominal group technique. Postal surveys may also be used as a means of identifying consensus (Penney et al, 1993). The advantage of the local consensus method is its convenience. It is quick and does not require the expertise needed to appraise research literature, and it is not surprising that it is the most common approach. The disadvantage is that the consensus group may overlook important research evidence, with the consequence that the participants in audit will be asked to implement inappropriate care. Given that the purpose of audit is to ensure that routine care complies with the best available evidence, this could be regarded as a fatal flaw. Also, when evidence is not used as the basis for criteria, there is a possibility that different consensus groups will come to different conclusions. In a study of the development of appropriateness ratings for surgical procedures conducted in Israel and the United Kingdom, panels composed of surgeons approved more indications than did panels containing a mixture of specialities (Fraser et al, 1994). There were also differences between the countries even when the composition of the panels was similar.

2.4   EVIDENCE-BASED CRITERIA

2.4.1   Principles

The criticisms of criteria developed through consensus can be avoided if formal methods are used to base them on the best available research evidence. Four principles for criteria of this type have been described (Baker and Fraser, 1995). First, they should be based on research evidence. Second, they should be prioritized. Some elements of care may be more important than others in that they have different impacts on outcome. Therefore, criteria for elements of care that have a major impact on outcome should be assigned a greater priority than those which have less impact. Furthermore, the strength of research evidence may also vary, and should be taken into account in prioritizing criteria. We classified those that are supported by strong research evidence and have an important impact on outcome as 'must do', those that have less impact on outcome or are supported by less good evidence as 'should do', and those which are only poorly supported by evidence as 'could do'.

Third, it should be possible to measure compliance with the criteria. Therefore, they should be worded to make clear exactly what data should be sought. Finally, criteria should be appropriate to the clinical setting in which they are to be used. For example, the criteria in an audit of the management of depression by general practitioners would be different to those in an audit of the same topic by clinical psychologists. Psychologists have the expertise to offer cognitive therapy and their audit might include several criteria about this treatment, but would not include detailed criteria about drug therapy.

2.4.2 Methods of development

A variety of methods has been used to develop evidence-based criteria. In a programme to develop measures of appropriateness for key medical and surgical procedures in the US, the findings of extensive literature reviews were submitted to carefully selected panels (Matchar et al, 1992). In the case of endarterectomy, for example, approximately 1800 articles were initially identified during the literature search. Those articles that did not meet certain predefined quality criteria or were not relevant were eliminated. Those retained were used to draw up an initial list of criteria, which was then submitted to the panel who were asked to rate on a numerical scale the appropriateness of each.

Whilst such a costly and labour intensive approach might be justified when developing criteria of appropriateness to be used by insurance companies to assess requests for reimbursements from providers in the USA, it would be impractical for professionally led clinical audit. With the arrival of new methods for collecting, appraising and summarizing research evidence, it is also becoming unnecessary. Efficient methods for developing criteria are now available. The most important advance has been the arrival of the systematic review.

A well conducted systematic review identifies all studies relevant to the topic in question, appraises the studies and selects only those of good quality. The data from these are extracted and synthesized, producing a conclusion made credible by the degree of underlying evidence. Although reviews of this type are an advance, they are not without problems. As new research is published, they become out of date; they require substantial time and resources to complete, and as the technology involved is new we are not yet fully aware of all the methodological weaknesses. However, despite these qualifications, systematic reviews are more likely to provide reliable summaries of evidence than are authoritative experts.

Clinical practice guidelines go one step further than reviews. For many clinical topics, evidence is limited or lacking altogether. Furthermore, the management of most conditions involves many clinical decisions, including those concerned with diagnosis, investigations, treatment choices and long term follow-up. It would be unusual for a single systematic review to be able to address all these concerns. A guideline can take into account the absence of evidence and the full range of issues in managing a particular condition. The starting point for a guideline is a systematic review of the literature, but a representative expert panel is also asked to provide recommendations based on that evidence, and where evidence is lacking to use its own best opinions. The best guidelines make clear which recommendations are supported by strong evidence and which are based largely on the opinion of the panel. This type of evidence-based guideline is an advance over the informal consensus methods used in the past, although as yet there is insufficient experience of their use for their potential weaknesses and adverse effects to be fully understood. For example, we need more information about the impact of the panel on the recommendations. It might be argued that when evidence is lacking, the individual practitioner in association with the patient should weigh up the options rather than a remote panel.

Guidelines may be used as the starting point for the development of review criteria. In the USA, methods have been devised by the Agency for Health Care Policy and Research (AHCPR) to develop criteria from its own guidelines (Hadorn et al, 1996). However, relatively few guidelines have undergone such rigorous development as those of the AHCPR. Before devising criteria, the quality of the source guidelines should be appraised (Cluzeau et al, 1995) and those found to be unsatisfactory should not be used.

An alternative to local selection of criteria is to employ systematically developed audit protocols. We have developed a method for devising evidence-based criteria, using either guidelines or systematic reviews as the starting point, leading to standard protocols that can be widely used (Fraser et al, 1997). This is described in outline in Box 2.3, but even though guidelines or reviews are used as the source point, detailed literature searching is still needed.

Audit of performance is one feature of the evidence-based medicine approach to clinical practice in which the practitioner is expected to be able to frame questions about clinical practice and use bibliographic databases to locate appropriate studies for appraisal in order to answer those questions (Sackett and Rosenberg, 1995). Although the selection of one or two criteria might be feasible using this approach, the systematic development of a comprehensive set for a particular condition would be demanding without recourse to good quality summaries of the literature such as systematic reviews of evidence-based guidelines or audit protocols.

Box 2.3   Development of evidence-based criteria (Fraser et al, 1997)

- Identify key elements of care from guidelines or systematic reviews.
- Undertake focused systematic reviews.
- Prioritize criteria.
- Prepare full documentation of the process.
- Submit criteria to peer review.

2.5   COLLECTING CONVINCING EVIDENCE ABOUT PERFORMANCE

The collection of data about current performance involves the use of basic epidemiological or research skills which should be readily understood by all health professionals. However, as our review of published audits revealed, errors are all too common. In planning data collection, a few simple rules should be followed (Box 2.4). We will illustrate them through selected case studies, identified in the review of audits (Table 2.2).

2.5.1   The patient population

Audit involves the collection of data about groups of patients, and the choice of which patients to include can substantially influence the findings. For example, the findings of an audit of major adverse events such as pulmonary embolus after surgery would appear flattering if certain patient groups such as the elderly were excluded. In assessing care in outpatient departments, patients who fail to attend follow-up appointments can present a particular problem. Some of them may have failed to attend because they were dissatisfied with the service and have decided to seek care privately; others may have experienced a

---

Box 2.4   Rules for data collections in audit

1. *The patient population*
- Types of patients to be stated.
- Patients involved identified.
- Equivalent patient populations in first and second data collections.

2. *Samples (if used)*
- Representative.
- Size calculated and adequate.
- Equivalent samples in both data collections.

3. *Data extraction*
- Explicit data extraction rules used.
- When more than one extractor used, data extraction is tested for inter-rater reliability.

4. *Data analysis*
- The proportion of cases which comply with each criterion is calculated.
- When samples have been used confidence intervals are calculated.

deterioration in their condition and been admitted to another hospital. Diabetes is a common topic for audit in primary care, but some patients may not be recorded in the practice diabetes register. These patients may be at particular risk because they do not make full use of available health care.

Misleading findings can also be caused by including patients who should have been excluded. It is possible that some patients classified as having a particular disease actually do not have the disease, or to have a less serious condition. In assessing care of patients with breast cancer, the mistaken inclusion of patients with benign breast disorders would give a false impression of the outcome of care. If healthy patients mistakenly thought to have diabetes are included in a diabetes audit, information about their blood sugar control will appear remarkably good.

A third problem arises from the need to undertake a second data collection. By the time this takes place, there may have been changes in the patient population; for example, the average age of patients admitted to a coronary care unit may have increased, patients with colorectal cancer may now be referred at an earlier stage of disease, or more people with type II diabetes may have been diagnosed as a result of a concerted screening policy. In these circumstances, differences between the findings from the first and second data collections might be entirely due to changes in the patient population.

Steps can be taken to avoid these problems. To ensure that all patients are identified, several patient registers can be used and compared to each other, as in the audits described in Boxes 2.5 and 2.6. A clear definition of the types of patient to include is essential, such as all children aged 0–16 (Box 2.7). It may be helpful to include a set of criteria that must be fulfilled for the diagnosis of the condition to be confirmed. Those patients who cannot be shown to meet the diagnostic criteria can then be excluded. Special efforts may be required to track down patients who fail to return for follow-up, beginning with seeking information about deaths and admissions. To avoid problems due to changes in the patient population, the second data collection should not be delayed too long. If seasonal factors influence case mix, as in respiratory infections, the second data collection should take place at the same time of the year as the first. Should the population change despite these precautions, it may be necessary to modify the analysis to highlight those types of patients that were comparable to those in the first data collection.

2.5.2   Samples

When the number of patients is relatively small, sampling is not required (see Boxes 2.5 and 2.6), but often there are so many patients that sampling is unavoidable. Sometimes, patients to be included are identified through events

Box 2.5 An audit of notifications, audiological referrals and chemoprophylaxis of contacts in meningitis in children

In the management of meningitis, several elements of care not directly related to acute treatment are important, but may be overlooked. Therefore, an audit was undertaken in a single children's hospital (Shields et al, 1995). Criteria were selected for the notification of cases to local officers for communicable disease control, the administration of chemoprophylaxis to family and household contacts, and hearing assessments of recovered children. The standards of compliance for these criteria were that they should be fulfilled for all cases (i.e. the standards were set at 100%).

In collecting data, cases were identified from several sources to ensure that no case was missed. For each data collection, all patients with meningitis in a 12-month period were included. Data were collected from several types of records: the officers of communicable disease records, ward notification records, ward drug records, case notes, and the audiology department computer. In the first 12 months, 36 patients were identified, in the second 12 months there were 32. There were improvements in the level of compliance with the criteria, a conclusion supported by the findings of Chi square tests. The methods used to implement change were feedback of the results to an audit meeting, agreement of actions to be taken, display of guidelines on ward notice boards, and circulation of written information about the policy to all relevant staff.

Box 2.6 An audit of breast examinations in women taking hormone replacement therapy

A general practitioner had been running a menopause clinic according to a clinical policy, recording details in a computer (Parry, 1993). The criterion chosen for the audit was that patients being prescribed hormone replacement therapy should have had a breast examination within the previous 6 months, a standard of 100% being set. Patients who were receiving hormone replacement therapy were identified by searching the computer and by a manual search of paper records. The computer data were incomplete, with more information being recorded in the paper records. Although the proportion of patients being examined was initially low, the second data collection confirmed that improvements had taken place. To implement change, a new system was introduced to recall patients, and the recording system was modified.

Box 2.7   An audit of delays before emergency surgery

Delays are one cause of avoidable morbidity associated with emergency operations. This audit was undertaken to address this problem (Galland and Dehn, 1995). The patients included were those who underwent emergency surgery during periods of 2 months for each data collection. The first data collection indicated a median delay for appendicectomies of 280 min, and 111 min for perforated duodenal ulcer. For all types of conditions combined, the median delay was 225 min. At the second data collection, the delay for appendicectomies had fallen to 89 min, perforated duodenal ulcer to nil, and for all conditions combined it was 75 min. A Mann–Whitney test was used to assess the statistical significance of these changes. To implement improvements, a dedicated emergency theatre was introduced, available throughout the working day.

Box 2.8   The recording of childhood accidental injury information in primary care

Accidents are common in childhood, and it has been argued that some might be prevented if primary health care teams could identify children at increased risk and intervene. Eight general practices took part in this audit (Marsh et al, 1995). Random samples of general practitioner and practice/clinic nurse records of children aged 0–16 in these practices were reviewed to extract data about recording of accidents and their nature. The results were fed back to the practice teams in written reports and practice-based feedback discussions. After the first data collection, improvements took place, for example the type of accident was recorded in 72%. The statistical significance was assessed with Chi square tests.

such as referrals or admissions rather than from a stable population listed on a disease register. Therefore, one approach is to include all those patients presenting during a defined period of time (see Box 2.7). A problem with this method is that it is difficult to predict with certainty the eventual number of patients, and the type of patient may differ between data collections. In the example in Box 2.7, there was a small decline in the total number of patients identified in the second data collection; in particular, there were fewer cases of appendicectomy. This was handled in the analysis by calculating data according to type of condition. Another weakness with period samples is ensuring that sufficient numbers of patients are included to ensure confidence in the findings. It can be helpful to determine the total number of patients likely to present over a long period, such as year. It would then be possible to calculate a satisfactory sample size from the total annual 'population'. When large numbers of patients are involved, sampling is required, and random samples are most likely to result in a sample that does accurately indicate care given to the population as a whole. Random sampling was employed in the audit described in Box 2.7. It is simple to generate random numbers from a random numbers table in a statistics textbook (Campbell and Machin, 1993) or by using a pocket calculator. There are very few occasions when the use of a random sample is impossible, but when it is, systematic samples offer a reasonable alternative.

Whenever samples are used, there is a danger that error will be introduced. It is impossible to be absolutely certain that the findings from a sample of patients do accurately represent information about the population as a whole, but it is possible to reduce the degree of likely error to a reasonable minimum. Provided the sample is random, the calculation of the required sample size takes into account the degree of risk of error that is acceptable. Whilst methods to calculate sample sizes may appear complicated, in audit they are relatively simple (see, for example, Jarvis, 1997a).

2.5.3 Data extraction

Clinical records are the most common source of data in audit, but records cannot contain the details of every element of care. Health professionals select which items to record, and when the audit is concerned with topics not likely to be recorded, other methods of data collection will be needed. For example, observation may be required in audits of communications between professional and patient. Even information about an element of care that is more likely to be recorded is sometimes omitted because the professional is too busy, or the notes are missing. In these circumstances, it is not possible confidently to assume that the absence of a record indicates an omission in care. However, alternative records are sometimes available, as in the audit in Box 2.6 in which both computer and manual prescribing records were used. Another approach is to ask patients to report on the content of care.

Two people extracting data may interpret the content of a set of records in different ways. When an entry is illegible, one person might decide the data are missing, another might try to guess the meaning of the text. If the records are extensive, one data extractor might search through them diligently, another may be less painstaking and miss some items of information. Even when the same information is legible and found by both extractors, it may be interpreted in different ways. For example, an entry of 'BP' followed by a tick might be assumed by one data extractor to mean that the blood pressure had been checked and was normal, but another extractor might decide that it meant that the blood pressure had been checked, but the result may have been either normal or abnormal. Problems of this type can be addressed by the preparation of an explicit set of data extraction instructions. It is also possible to check the reliability of data collection by comparing the findings of two collectors using the same small sample of notes. The level of agreement between the collectors can be expressed as a percentage, and low levels of agreement would indicate that the data are probably unreliable.

2.5.4   Data analysis

In audit, data analysis is generally simple. Provided that samples were not used, all that is required is to determine the proportion of patients whose care was in compliance with the criteria. Tests of the statistical significance of changes in performance between data collections are not required as there is no intention of generalizing the findings beyond the included patients to a wider population. For a whole population, the changes are actual, and not estimates. Therefore, there is no test for significance, and there is no error due to sampling.

However, when samples have been used statistical analysis is employed to take into account the possibility of error when inferring that the findings of the sample represent the true level of care of the population as a whole. In our examples, Chi square or similar tests were used. However, confidence intervals are preferable as they provide more meaningful information to participants in audit. The calculation of confidence intervals for the data usually collected in audit is straight forward using a pocket calculator and an elementary under-standing of arithmetic (Gardner and Altman, 1989; Jarvis, 1997b).

2.6   SUMMARY POINTS

- Since many audits have methodological weaknesses such as poor criteria, inadequate samples and failure to complete the cycle, it is not surprising that change often does not occur.
- Convincing research evidence about appropriate care is the starting point for audit.
- Practical methods are available for developing evidence-based criteria for audit, including the use of existing systematic reviews and guidelines, specific audit protocols, and direct use of research literature employing the skills of evidence-based medicine.
- Objective evidence about current performance is also needed. To achieve this, the patient population must be complete. If samples are used, they should be representative and of adequate size. Data extraction should be standardized and follow explicit rules.

REFERENCES

Baker R and Fraser RC (1995) Development of review criteria: linking guideline and quality assessment. *BMJ* **311**:370–373.

Baker R, Hearnshaw H, Robertson N, Cooper A and Cheater F (1995a) Assessing the work of medical audit advisory groups in promoting audit in general practice. *Quality in Health Care* **4**:234–239.

Baker R, Robertson N and Farooqi A (1995b) Audit in general practice: factors influencing participation. *BMJ* **311**:31–34.

Black NA and Thompson EM (1993) Medical audit, the views of junior doctors. *Journal of Management in Medicine* **7**:33–42.

Buttery Y, Walshe K, Coles J and Bennett J (1994) *The Development of Audit. Findings of a National Survey of Healthcare Provider Units in England*. London: Caspe Research.

Campbell MJ and Machin D (1993) *Medical Statistics. A Common-sense Approach*. Chichester: John Wiley & Sons.

Cluzeau F, Littlejohns P, Grimshaws J and Feder G (1995) Draft appraisal instrument for clinical guidelines. In: Royal College of General Practitioners, *The Development and Implementation of Clinical Guidelines*. Report from practice 26. London: Royal College of General Practitioners.

Fraser GM, Pilpel D et al (1994) Effect of panel composition on appropriateness ratings. *International Journal of Quality in Health Care* **6**:251–255.

Fraser RC, Khunti K, Baker R and Lakhani M (1997) Effective audit in general practice: a method for systematically developing audit protocols containing evidence-based review criteria. *Br J Gen Pract* **47**:743–746.

Galland RB and Dehn TCB (1995) Emergency operating theatres for general surgical emergencies a prospective audit. *Medical Audit News* **5**:139–140.

Gardner MJ and Altman DG (1989) *Statistics with Confidence. Confidence Intervals and Statistical Guidelines*. London: British Medical Journal.

Hadorn DC, Baker DW, Kamberg CJ and Brooks RH (1996) Phase II of the AHCPR – sponsored heart failure: translating practice recommendations into review criteria. *Joint Commission Journal on Quality Improvement* **22**:265–276.

Hearnshaw H, Baker R and Cooper A (1998) A survey of audit activity in general practice. *Br J Gen Pract* **48**:979–981.

Hopkins A (1996) Clinical audit: time for a reappraisal? *J R Coll Phys* **30**:415–425.

Jarvis P (1997a) Choosing the correct sample size: how large is large? *Audit Trends* **5**: 141–143.

Jarvis P (1997b). Describing the results of audit, is average enough? *Audit Trends* **5**:25–27.

Lembcke PA (1956) Medical auditing by scientific methods, illustrated by major female pelvic surgery. *JAMA* **162**:646–655.

Marsh P, Kendrick D and Williams EI (1995) The impact of audit on the recording of childhood accidental injury information by primary healthcare teams. *Audit Trends* **3**:47–52.

Matchar DB, Golstein LB, McCrory DC et al (1992) *Carotid Endartrectomy: a Literature Review and Ratings of Appropriateness*. Santa Monica, CA: Rand. Rand JRA-05.

Parry JM (1993) Hormone replacement therapy and breast cancer. *Medical Audit News* **3**:105–106.

Penney GC, Glasier A and Templeton A (1993) Agreeing criteria for audit of the management of induced abortion: an approach by national consensus survey. *Quality in Health Care* **2**:167–169.

Sackett DL and Rosenberg WMC (1995) The need for evidence-based medicine. *J R Soc Med* **88**:620–624.

Shields MD, Adams D, Beresford P and Dodge JA (1995) Managing meningitis in children: audit of notification, rifampicin prophylaxis, and audio logical referrals. *Quality in Health Care* **4**:268–272.

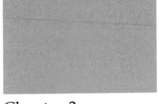

Chapter 3

A SYSTEMATIC APPROACH TO MANAGING CHANGE

Noelle Robertson

The times they are a changing – Bob Dylan

Audit and the wider drive towards clinical effectiveness have been accompanied by a growing and often unwelcome realization that death is no longer the only certainty. Change, particularly visible through the restructuring of the NHS, would appear to be an inevitable and integral part of 1990s health care. Since health professionals must now offer care based on evidence of its effectiveness, many have found that they must alter or stop well-established patterns of behaviour and adopt new ones. A not uncommon refrain of the health professional is that whilst change was all right once, it has gone on too long (with apologies to Ogden Nash).

Of course, the processes of change and audit are intimately linked. In setting standards and measuring performance, audit is specifically geared to identifying aspects of care that may need modification. The central premise of this book is that successful audit and successful change go hand in hand. However, whilst change, either to undertake audit or to respond to the findings of audit, might be desirable and necessary, implementation can be a complex and at times difficult process (Haines and Jones, 1994). It was Fowkes (1982) who observed that just because audit identifies a need to change, there is no guarantee that a change will follow. The difficulties that have been experienced in completing the audit cycle and making change have caused a re-evaluation of how change can be most readily achieved.

3.1 A BRIEF HISTORY

Earlier efforts to update and shape professional practice have relied heavily upon continuing professional education and the provision of new information on better ways of working (via conferences, lectures and workshops). However,

Implementing Change With Clinical Audit. Edited by Richard Baker, Hilary Hearnshaw and Noelle Robertson.
© 1999 John Wiley & Sons, Ltd.

current attempts to change professionals' behaviour are no longer guided solely by such formal continuing professional development activity which, alone, is relatively ineffective (Davis et al, 1995). Simply because a change in behaviour has inherent logic and benefit does not mean it will be adopted. We only have to ruefully re-examine some of our personal resolutions to reduce stress and improve health to recognize that even small and discrete changes to diet, alcohol or exercise regimes, although advisable, can be difficult to execute and sustain.

The relative lack of behaviour change resulting from educational programmes (Mazzuca, 1986; Kanouse and Jaccoby, 1988; Greco and Eisenberg, 1993), the limited impact of simple information transfer, and the realization that professionals do not progress linearly from the acquisition of knowledge through attitude change to altered behaviour, caused a re-evaluation of how change should be stimulated and encouraged. If education does not foster change, and knowledge is necessary but not sufficient, what other influences shape professional behaviour? To answer this question, a number of alternative strategies have been offered as solutions. These include clinical guidelines, reminders, feedback, sanctions and educational outreach (see Chapter 1).

However, the provision of these solutions is not sufficient to promote change. Oxman and colleagues' (1995) review emphasized the lack of a 'magic bullet', and no single strategy or solution will inevitably produce change in all health settings and for all topics. In the absence of predictably effective strategies to encourage professional behaviour change, what can we currently do to ensure that audit and other tools to improve quality have maximum impact? In short, this chapter encourages the reader to be analytical, reflective and systematic in approaching change. Because of the dearth of conclusive evidence to guide the choice of effective strategies, this chapter attempts to dissuade readers from opting for strategies that are simply familiar or available.

Instead, I will suggest how we can all become more effective change agents – by engaging in systematic attempts to understand and address the factors that influence change. Emphasis is placed on a clear analysis of the issues as an essential prerequisite before applying any implementation strategy. This means first identifying and defining any problems or obstacles impeding change before rushing to a solution. The chapter will also show that obstacles to change can be tackled systematically, with flexible use of theories to both understand obstacles and to help select strategies to overcome them. The relevance of this tailored approach to change will be illustrated with a more detailed examination of some useful psychological theories. The chapter will not, however, provide the reader with in-depth theoretical knowledge for identifying obstacles, but some additional reading and sources of advice are suggested at the end.

3.2 TO EVERY ACTION THERE MUST BE AN EQUAL AND OPPOSITE REACTION (Newton's Third Law)

Many specialists in organizational development and management studies describe change as a response to pressures. Some pressures act for (levers) and some against the change (obstacles or resistances), and may act synergistically or antagonistically (Warr, 1996). Pressures for change may be internal. For example, individuals or teams may be dissatisfied with the way they work or wish to improve their effectiveness. Pressures may also be externally generated. Technological advances are one source of external pressures, for example progress in computing which promotes the development of electronic clinical records. The external social climate can also create pressures, such as changing patient expectations which may shape the way health professionals conduct consultations and provide information. Additional external pressures include political ideology such as that which underpinned the internal market; and also audit, acting as an impetus for change by identifying strengths and weaknesses of care.

However, just as there are forces acting to promote change, there are also forces resisting change. These have been identified in professionals undertaking audit (Baker et al, 1995), with inadequate time and resources being most frequently cited. Other obstacles are commonly identified (Manchester Open Learning, 1993). Poor communication within an organization or team, a bureaucratic structure which stifles innovation, and fuzzy or competing management objectives can all hinder changes in organizations. Resistances which we personally experience may include reluctance to disrupt a comfortable routine, fear (of the unknown, of the consequences of a change or that any new demands will exceed our abilities), self-interest and a lack of any perceived benefits in changing. There is no uniform term to describe resistances or barriers. In this book, we intend to use obstacles as an umbrella term which may encompass both, and which implies that they can be overcome.

Resistance or obstacles to change are often labelled pejoratively. Yet change, even when benefit is the likely outcome, can be a profoundly unsettling experience. It is likely that we can all identify recent changes in working practice that were accompanied by some trepidation at the prospect of altering what was familiar. Resistance is not necessarily a bad thing, but reflects a human comfort with the *status quo*, and we need to recognize it as an integral part of the change process. In order to encourage successful change, we must capitalize on, and utilize the pressures and levers for change, tackle the obstacles and in so doing shift the *status quo*. A necessary first step is, therefore, clearly to identify and delineate obstacles and levers before considering how best to address them.

Attempts to change professional behaviour have slowly acknowledged the prevalence of obstacles to change. Grol and Wensing (1995) explicitly examined general practitioners' perceived obstacles to implementing quality assurance activities including audit. Most prominent amongst these were lack of time, colleagues' negative attitudes to quality assurance, and anxiety about being scrutinized and criticized by peers. Other studies have elicited similar obstacles as professionals attempt to incorporate research findings in daily practice (Closs and Cheater, 1996).

Other studies have explored the positive pressures or levers for change. Armstrong et al (1996) interviewed 18 general practitioners about their reasons for changes in prescribing behaviour over the previous 6 months. They identi- fied three levers promoting change. The first was accumulation, there being no single trigger to change but a growing body of disparate evidence from opinion leaders, peers and journal articles. The second was a challenge to clinical prac- tice through significant events such as a patient death or the unexpected success of a therapeutic regime, confounding the doctor's expectations. The third was the process of continuity – change occurred because it was congruent with current practice such as an accepted need to rein in prescribing costs. Similarly, diverse pressures for change have also been outlined by Allery et al (1997). Using a critical incident technique, she studied the factors which doctors in primary and secondary care settings described as changing their practice. Change again resulted from a combination of factors, particularly organizational such as management and staffing, and contact with other health professionals.

3.3   FRAMEWORKS TO FACILITATE CHANGE

Given that obstacles and levers exist, and that they may vary for different professionals in different environments and at different times, some form of categorization is useful both to organize knowledge and rationalize the use of strategies. Several authors have suggested that change strategies are likely to have more impact if targeted at particular settings where specific issues or circumstances may prevail, and have developed conceptual frameworks to support their arguments (Rogers, 1983; Grol, 1992).

Rogers described how innovations such as audit are adopted by professionals over a period of time, and categorized individuals by their willingness to take up new practices and procedures – from innovators, early adopters, early majority, late majority and laggards. These individuals can be plotted on the S-shaped curve (Stocking, 1992) depicting how an innovation is adopted over time (see Figure 3.1), and Rogers, along with others (Haines and Jones, 1994; Haines, 1996), have stressed that change strategies should be appropriate to the health professionals' position on this curve.

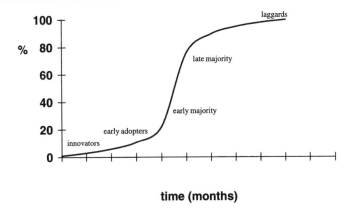

time (months)

Figure 3.1 The curve of innovation, showing the percentage of people adopting an innovation over time (Stocking, 1992)

Grol (1992) adapted this classification system to describe potential obstacles to change that might be influencing early adopters, the majority, or late adopters amongst general practitioners. From this, he too suggested that different strategies might be used at different stages of the adoption process. Within his framework, he suggested that early adopters, who are amenable to innovations such as audit, might need only facilitative measures such as education to change practice. Late adopters who faced obstacles might require more coercive strategies such as sanctions or legislation. Funk et al (1991) have offered similar perspectives in describing how new procedures are adopted by nurses, devising a tool to explore nurses' obstacles to using research findings.

Other authors have drawn more widely in developing frameworks to examine pressures for and against change. In the context of guideline implementation, Lomas (1994) developed a co-ordinated model to help understand the factors influencing guideline adoption. Integrating four approaches to changing clinical practice – social influence theory, diffusion of innovation literature, marketing and educational theories, Lomas' framework helps to provide a fuller picture of factors that can act at different times or together to help or hinder change. However, whilst both the Grol and Lomas frameworks show the need to consider diverse influences and strategies, only the former suggests that the obstacles must first be analysed. Neither suggest explicitly how obstacles might be assessed and strategies then selected.

We have developed a framework in which there is an explicit attempt to link the analysis of obstacles with specific implementation strategies using theories explaining behaviour change (Robertson et al, 1996). The framework makes no claims to be a complete model, nor does it encompass all theories of behaviour change. We have quite deliberately chosen theories which can help select strategies from a fairly circumscribed menu of interventions and omitted those which, although they may help identify obstacles, do not suggest ways of overcoming them. However, it provides a systematic basis for using our current understanding of human behaviour both to identify obstacles or levers to change in any situation and select strategies with the best chance of addressing them.

In doing this, we compare the assessment of obstacles to change and selection of implementation strategies with the diagnosis and management of symptoms of disease. To make sense of an array of patient symptoms, health professionals will refer to bodies of knowledge (i.e. theories) about health, illness and disease. This will help them to understand what the symptoms mean and guide them as they search for additional signs to further formulate what is happening, or to confirm a diagnosis. Theories can also indicate which treatment is likely to be of most benefit. For example, a patient who has recently been involved in a road traffic accident may present with distressing flashbacks to the event. Drawing on theory on the impact of trauma, the clinician may check for the presence of intrusive thoughts and avoidant behaviour that would suggest post-traumatic stress disorder. If the diagnosis is confirmed, the patient may be offered desensitization therapy, also derived from trauma theory, which should address and alleviate the symptoms.

Because the framework is designed to help change human behaviour, we use psychological theories which can describe and explain the attitudes, beliefs and behaviour of health professionals. Psychological theories can be loosely grouped by the level at which they explain behaviour change. Some theories focus on the individual health professional behaviour [for example Bandura's (1986) self-efficacy theory or Worden's (1991) model describing the consequences of loss – see Box 3.1]; others examine group behaviour (social comparison, social facilitation, 'groupthink' – see Box 3.2) of teams in primary, secondary and community settings; and yet others examine organizational behaviour (system theories, management theories – see Box 3.3) such as the operation of trusts, commissioning bodies and the NHS itself.

Our framework uses selected theories from these three categories to link obstacles and levers to change with strategies that the theories predict will be most effective. To illustrate the potential of the framework, emphasis will be placed on obstacles since these can often create more concern in attempts to change, particularly because they may appear difficult to identify. Furthermore, in most audits the levers are already operating, for example through the support of professionals to the choice of topic, participation in treatment, or funds provided to facilitate the audit. However, in a complete formulation of the factors influencing change, strategies should also be tailored to take advantage of levers.

As Tables 3.1–3.3 demonstrate, with familiar examples drawn from quality improvement, when change is not happening, it is possible to suggest what

Box 3.1 Psychological theories – individual behaviour

Self-efficacy (Bandura, 1986)

According to Bandura, behaviour change is determined by the beliefs an individual holds about their personal control. If a person feels able to solve a problem or undertake a particular task, they will feel more inclined to do so. High levels of self-efficacy – a belief in success – predict greater persistence and ultimate success in behaviours such as audit.

Mourning loss (Worden, 1987)

Worden describes a process of mourning following loss or bereavement. He argues that loss is emotionally destabilizing and that in order to re-establish equilibrium, an individual must address four tasks.

i)   Accepting the reality of the loss (and accepting that the practitioner you thought you were is gone).
ii) To experience the pain of grief.
iii) To adjust to a new you or environment.
iv) To withdraw emotional energy (from the practitioner you were) and invest it in the practitioner you now are.

Social influence theory (Zimbardo and Leippe, 1991)

Social influence is used to encompass processes where the behaviour of another has the effect, or intention, of changing how another person behaves, feels or thinks about something, and includes the effects of group norms and culture on behaviour.

might be preventing it (the obstacles), why that might be (the theories), and choose strategies that the theories predict will tackle the obstacles. Table 3.1 shows an individual professional who is not following a protocol or guideline. Psychological theories can offer a number of suggestions as to why that might be. If the professional is unsure whether they possess the knowledge or skills to apply the guideline recommendations, Bandura's construct of self-efficacy may be helpful (Box 3.1). It would suggest that since the professional is not confident that they can execute the behaviour requested in the guideline, then in order to comply they need to believe they can do what is needed (increasing efficacy expectations). The theory predicts that strategies that enhance efficacy expectations, such as training in requisite skills, information on how to undertake tasks suggested by the guideline, or positive feedback on current performance, are more likely to encourage change than those strategies which do not address the lack of self belief, such as simple dissemination of the guideline. Additionally, there may be strategies that the theory would suggest might be counter-

---

Box 3.2   Psychological theories – group behaviour

Social facilitation (Zajonc, 1965)

Early experiments in social psychology demonstrated how the presence of others in a working context could enhance performance on various tasks. The inverse of this phenomenon has also been shown in groups. If groups undertake audit in which there is no clear delineation of tasks, responsibility is diffused and performance is adversely affected.

Social influence and conformity (Moscovici, 1985)

When we are in a group and are asked to make an evaluation or judgement, we may find we disagree with the majority of the group members. If we decide that the majority view is more valid, we may change our evaluation, fearing we may be seen as less competent than the others. However, the majority view does not always prevail, and Moscovici sought an explanation for the impact of a powerful minority. Undertaking a series of experiments, he showed that a minority view would prevail if members had a pre-existing powerful role in the group and argued a consistent position with confidence. The power of the minority can be dispelled if the majority seek out allies with status and views consistent with developing norms.

Groupthink (Janis, 1972)

Janis, after reviewing political decision making, described groupthink – a phenomenon in groups where errors of judgement arise as a consequence of an extreme need for consensus. This is more likely to occur in very cohesive groups which feel threatened, and may be characterized by an over-optimistic view of the group's performance, pressures on dissenters, silence about any individual doubts and rationalizations to defend previous decisions or behaviour.

---

productive, such as feedback showing poor performance, which may diminish self-efficacy still further.

However, the professional may not have adopted the guideline recommendations because they are not ready to change. A theoretical interpretation is provided by the transtheoretical model (Prochaska et al, 1992) which will be described more fully later in the chapter. In essence, this theory categorizes professionals in a continuum from precontemplation (not considering change) to maintenance (consolidating changes in practice), and suggests that if a professional is content with current practice (a precontemplator), training is unlikely to promote change because it does not address the primary obstacle. In order to shift the professional closer to changing, that is starting to accept that

Box 3.3   Organizational theories

Power (Handy, 1993)

Handy pulls together a number of studies of sources of power in organizations and how they influence methods of change. He identifies a number of power sources which must first be identified before deciding on change strategies, for example:

- expert (power devised from recognized expertise);
- personal (charisma);
- negative (capacity to wreck change);
- position (resulting from role in the organization).

Culture (Harrison, 1972)

Culture refers not just to an ideology, but also to an implicit set of norms often described as 'the way we do things around here'. He describes four main types of culture – power, role, task and person. He argues that before embarking on a change strategy the prevailing culture should be identified and strategies tailored accordingly.

change is warranted, strategies such as feedback may be more appropriate, as they cause the professional to face current practice, disturbing the *status quo*, and increasing consideration of change. It is important to note from these examples that the same strategy may be indicated and effective in one situation but not in another, its effectiveness being determined by the obstacle present and its success in addressing it.

Individual obstacles and theories may not always relate to the rational nature of health professionals. A failure to adopt a guideline may be symptomatic of a professional resisting the evidence that they are not providing excellent care. One theory that helps to understand this resistance is the reaction to loss [the pain of losing the image of oneself as a competent professional, Worden (1991)]. The theory suggests that feedback showing inadequacies would simply exacerbate the emotional reaction and make change less likely. A more fruitful strategy would be to permit the expression of the professional's feelings through the provision of confidential and facilitated peer review. This would allow a safe context in which to express initial shock and denial, and share experiences with others, enabling a degree of acceptance before considering how improvement could be achieved.

Alternatively, the guideline may not be adopted because its source is seen to be compromised, for example if it has been produced by a group with vested interests. Since social influence theory (see Box 3.1) suggests that messages

Table 3.1 Framework for integrated obstacles to change, theory and strategies for change: the personal level (Robertson et al, 1996)

Observed behaviour	Obstacle	Theory	Strategies	
			More effective	Less effective
Doctor not following a clinical practice guideline	Thinks he or she lacks knowledge/ability	Self-efficacy	Involvement in guideline development Practical support and training	Dissemination alone
	Practitioner unwilling to consider change (thinks current practice is good enough)	Preparedness to change	Feedback showing poor performance	Feedback showing poor performance Practical support and training
	Source of guidelines perceived to be not reputable	Social influence	Endorsement by respected opinion leader with no likely gain to self	Endorsement by group with commercial or political interest
	Denial (of evidence of performance deficiency)	Bereavement reaction	Provision of safe and facilitated setting to admit deficiencies	Publication of performance league tables

Table 3.2 Framework for integrating obstacles to change, theory and strategies for change: the group level (Robertson et al, 1996)

Observed behaviour	Obstacle	Theory	Strategies	
			More effective	Less effective
A multisite audit has been organized but a health care team has failed to change clinical behaviour	Team members think that others will undertake the audit or change, so do nothing (social loafing and free riding)	Inverse social facilitation	Assign individuals with identifiable responsibilities for the change and make each accountable	General education about how to effect changes
	Powerful minority of team think that change is unnecessary	Social comparison	Introduce a few people with status and expertise to ally with less powerful team members	Suggest junior member of staff be responsible for implementing change
	Team spirit and morale are high; and opinion is that performance is very good	Groupthink	Use of respected outsiders to challenge team ideas	Exhorting team to change behaviour

Table 3.3 Framework for integrating obstacles to change, theory and strategies for change: the organizational level (Robertson et al, 1996)

Observed behaviour	Obstacle	Theory	Strategies	
			More effective	Less effective
Failure to implement national recommendations about use of an equally effective but less expensive treatment	Doctors reject the role of managers in discussing clinical issues	Power theory	Change power relation	Exhortation
	Doctors do not appreciate the consequences of the expensive treatment for the service or for colleagues	Cultural change	Doctor helped to perceive the problem from colleagues and managers' perspective	Management edict

such as guidelines will be responded to more favourably if they have been developed by credible and respected experts or institutions. Endorsement by an opinion leader is also likely to encourage adoption more readily than that of a politically or commercially compromised source.

Because health professionals seldom work in isolation, it is also important to consider obstacles (and pertinent theories) that may be relevant to groups. Table 3.2 uses the example/symptom of an organized multisite audit in which a team of professionals has failed to implement indicated changes. One possible obstacle is that team members each believe that someone else will implement the changes and therefore absolve themselves of responsibility. This can be interpreted as an act of inverse social facilitation (see Box 3.2) – little benefit will be derived from a strategy that treats the team collectively with general information on change. A strategy much more likely to facilitate the change will be one that allocates specific roles and tasks to team members, clarifying responsibilities and countering the belief that someone else will undertake the tasks.

Other possible obstacles include the presence and power of a minority in a team who feel that change is unnecessary. Despite being numerically greater, the less powerful majority may feel that they have to comply; for example, a ward team may not feel able to challenge the authority of the consultant. Such an obstacle can be tackled using theory on conformity (Box 3.2), which argues that the influence of the powerful minority can be overcome if the majority can ally themselves with others who have status and/or expertise in the areas of contention. This is likely to prove more effective than the all too frequent strategy of delegating responsibility for implementation to a junior team member. This delegation may diffuse the tension in the team, but is unlikely to produce meaningful change.

But it is not just dysfunctional teams that may have difficulty changing. An often overlooked obstacle within a group is extremely positive team spirit. Such teams may resist change because they believe their care is optimal. They are often identified by firm, respected leadership and powerful cohesion. The theory of groupthink suggests that cohesion and the need to be a member of a team is so strong that dissent is suppressed and self-criticism diminished. Groupthink would suggest that requests to change practice would be perceived as confrontational, and that cohesion would increase in response to such an attack. In order to reduce groupthink and free up expressions of discontent, strategies to consider would be those in which respected outsiders could provide support to those who feel the group may be wrong but are fearful of being ostracized, should they voice their concerns.

There are fewer psychological theories that have direct relevance to obstacles occurring in organizations. However, the fields of both organizational development and management science have useful explanatory theories, and although not included in this chapter, sociological and economic theories may also be considered.

Table 3.3 outlines the possible obstacles underpinning an organization's failure to reduce use of an expensive treatment when a cheaper, and equally safe and effective alternative is available. One obstacle may be that clinicians have ignored management pressure to adopt the new treatment because they believe that since managers are not clinically expert they cannot adequately judge subtle clinical issues. Clinicians are therefore exerting their expert power to diminish and reject management advice (Box 3.3). Such a theoretical interpretation would suggest that further management pressure would be ineffective, whereas a renegotiation of the manager–clinician relationship, particularly giving management more power and credibility, might encourage change.

Alternatively the obstacle may be that clinicians are not sensitive to the impact of their costly behaviour on the organization and its constituent parts. Management edicts are likely only to reinforce isolation and the failure to comprehend the needs of colleagues. If the obstacle is interpreted as a facet of the organizational culture, then a change in that culture may be more effective. In this approach, professionals may be encouraged to consider the impact of their behaviour on others through, for example, shadowing, more effective communication strategies or re-engineering the process of care so that professionals can see more readily what different disciplines contribute.

3.4 HOW TO USE THE FRAMEWORK

This framework is designed primarily to direct the choice of implementation strategies in a rational, systematic way, guided by what is already known about human behaviour. But how should it be used? To use the framework, we suggest that it is important to apply science to the process of facilitating change. This means that the selection of strategies should be governed by scientific method. There should be clear descriptions of the obstacles and levers to change, the construction of alternative hypotheses as to why these are present, informed by psychological knowledge, and testing of the hypotheses by tracking the effects of any strategies used. Even where extensive theoretical knowledge is not available, hypotheses can still be generated about why change does or does not occur using experience and qualitative judgements (this is discussed further in Chapter 4).

What is meant by generating a number of hypotheses? In the framework, a number of alternative obstacles are suggested to explain why change was not occurring. These are essentially hypotheses about the reasons for the behaviour that is observed and are based upon detailed initial observations. It is important to generate a number of initial hypotheses for a variety of reasons: (i) to avoid focusing prematurely on one obstacle and ignoring equally valid obstacles which would provide a complete picture; (ii) to try to minimize subjective views or preconceptions that could bias the perception of what is occurring; (iii) to help simplify the often complex and conflicting information about what is impeding change.

Having generated these working hypotheses, they need to be defined in such a way that they can be tested and theory used to select the implementation strategy. The consequences of the selected intervention(s) are then monitored in audit by assessing the degree of change, if any, and from subjective reports by those who have experienced the strategy. This process, termed progressive hypothesizing, is outlined in Table 3.4. The approach is implicit in applied psychological practice and embodies an assumption that professionals involved in understanding and managing behaviour change will use and evaluate strategies for change through applied research, that is be both scientists and practitioners (Barlow et al, 1986).

This progressive approach is both systematic and objective, and emphasizes not only rigorous information gathering, but also constant evaluation of a strategy's impact. It stresses that efforts to change professional practice should be driven by a continual assessment of the assumptions and theories underpinning the strategies used as well as continuous scrutiny of the behaviour that is or is not changing. Since attempts to change behaviour may themselves produce unforeseen obstacles, or the context may alter (the membership of a team may change, funding for audit may appear or local/national health priorities may evolve) this cyclical process is particularly relevant, since it can accommodate such changes.

3.5 NOTHING IS SO PRACTICAL AS A GOOD THEORY (Kurt Lewin)

The framework incorporates a number of theories that may be valuable to identify obstacles and suggest strategies to overcome them. However, not all readers may be familiar with the theories. In order to help familiarization with the process of diagnosing obstacles and tailoring implementation strategies to use within the work setting, one theory particularly relevant to individual behaviour change is discussed in more detail below. It has been selected because it shows considerable promise in understanding how current implementation strategies work, and may be helpful to shape and develop strategies in the future.

Table 3.4   Progressive hypothesizing

---

1. Initial assessment (what change is wanted, what change is occurring/failing to occur).
2. Provisional hypotheses (what are the likeliest/less likely obstacles/levers to change).
3. Gathering of additional information to support/refute hypotheses and prioritize obstacles.
4. Select strategy suggested by theory to have best chance of addressing obstacle(s).
5. Implement strategy(ies).
6. Monitor progress.
7. Revise hypotheses.
8. Assess outcome.

3.6   TRANSTHEORETICAL MODEL OF CHANGE

One of the most useful theories underpinning health behaviour change is the transtheoretical model, often more colloquially known as preparedness to change. Developed in the USA by Prochaska and DiClemente (1992), it has emerged and been validated from extensive work on the addictive behaviours, most particularly focusing on the process by which smokers stop smoking. It is increasingly being applied to understand the intentional behaviour of a variety of non-clinical populations, and may therefore be useful in considering intentional behaviours of health professionals (for example, agreement to take part in audit).

The central premise of the theory (so called because it encompasses stages of change common to a variety of psychological therapies) is that people change their behaviour not in an all or nothing fashion but through a series of incremental stages determined by their motivational state. Prochaska and DiClemente have identified five stages: (i) precontemplation, in which an individual has no intention to change; (ii) contemplation, in which change may be a possibility in the future (e.g. the next 6 months); (iii) preparation, in which there are explicit plans and activity focusing on change; (iv) action, in which a change occurs and (v) maintenance, in which any change in behaviour is consolidated. Successful change occurs as the individual proceeds through the stages, building on the preceding stage. This can take a long time, as progress may often be erratic, and attempts to change may fail, causing a return to the previous stage, rather like the game of snakes and ladders.

Those involved in audit, either as participants or facilitators, are likely to have experienced or witnessed these stages. Precontemplation is distinguished by a number of features, the main one of which is overt resistance. Precontemplators can often be defensive about their practice, because previous attempts to change have been unsuccessful, because they have little insight about their practice or because they believe there is little they can or need to do. In the case of agreeing to take part in audit, when faced with information about audit, precontemplators may respond by discounting the facts or excusing their own behaviour.

Contemplators, because they are thinking about changing what they do or the way they do it, may be more amenable to feedback generated by audit. However, they are unlikely to show commitment and will probably be weighing up the pros and cons of any change, as they have been doing for some time – the gestation period before any preparation for change can last up to 18 months. To illustrate this phenomenon, Prochaska et al (1992) cite an example described by Benjamin in 1987. Returning home one evening, Benjamin met a stranger who was lost and seeking directions. Having provided detailed directions, Benjamin became concerned when the stranger started to walk in the opposite direction and shouted that he should be heading the other way. The stranger replied that he was aware of where he should be going but was not quite ready – an archetypal contemplator.

People who are preparing to change are distinguished by their tentative steps towards change. Using our example of participation in audit, they may have contacted their local audit group or have attempted some preliminary data collection that would form the basis of an audit. Another distinctive feature of preparation is an explicit intention to undertake a project in the following month. Those who have progressed further and reached the stage of action have made some visible change to what they do, expending considerable effort in the process. Within the audit context, this will most probably be the completion of an audit cycle. And finally, those who are at the stage of maintaining their change will be continuing their audit efforts, perhaps consolidating the gains made from a previous cycle or moving to audit a new topic. Using this model, and identifying how motivated a professional is, can help decide what and whether an intervention is worthwhile.

However, the model includes another important and helpful feature. In addition to identifiable stages of change, Prochaska and DiClemente also describe transition processes occurring between one stage and the next. They argue that since different transition processes operate between the different stages (Table 3.5), then different types of implementation strategy are needed to encourage the shift from stage to stage. So for those not yet even contemplating change and who are not considering audit, consciousness raising via education about how audit is done and its benefits may be all that should be attempted to shift them towards contemplation. Observing how others have managed audit successfully or providing feedback on the professionals' own performance may shift those who are contemplating change to preparation, by allowing them to evaluate how they feel about the process.

Gaining the professional's commitment appears to be essential if people are to shift from preparation to action. Providing data collection sheets and offering to

Table 3.5 Strategies of change and suggested strategies and facilitate transition (from Prochaska and DiClemente, 1992)

Precontemplation	Contemplation	Preparation	Action	Maintenance
Raising awareness				
	Re-evaluating feelings about change			
			Increasing levels of commitment	
				Reinforcement of change

analyse audit data can structure and ease the process. Alternatively, getting participation in an organized audit is a useful 'foot in the door' technique. Having made a relatively small initial commitment to undertake a supported audit, when a bigger demand is made, perhaps being asked to complete their own audit, then the professional is more likely to comply. They now see themselves as someone who audits, is capable of doing so, and will shift from mere preparation to action.

Finally, once professionals have undertaken audits that have led to change in clinical practice, active strategies can still be used to ensure that the change is maintained. Prochaska and DiClemente argue that maintenance builds on each of the previous processes, and that successful strategies are those which reinforce the change in practice and prevent relapse. Reinforcement strategies may include, for example, non-financial rewards or reminders (such as newsletters) or continuing contact with audit facilitators.

The stages of change approach is relevant to the overall message of this chapter. The art of changing professional practice is slowly developing and as yet we cannot be certain about why some strategies fail when others succeed, either wholly or partially. However, we can become more systematic and reflective about how we attempt to change our own or others' behaviour. By using the framework described in this chapter in conjunction with progressive hypothesizing, we can help ourselves and others become active consumers of research and, through evaluating the effectiveness of change strategies that we ourselves employ, add to a growing body of knowledge on processes enhancing change.

3.7 SUMMARY POINTS

- Change in clinical practice or bahaviour is often the most difficult part of audit.

- Change can be enhanced by adopting a systematic approach in which obstacles and levers are clarified.
- Implementation strategics can be rationally selected by tailoring them to identified obstacles which have been clarified using explicit (and implicit) theories of human behaviour.
- A framework to link obstacles and strategies, via theories has been described. This can be used in conjunction with progressive hypothesizing.

REFERENCES

Allery LA, Owen PA and Robling MR (1997) Why general practitioners and consultants change their clinical practice: a critical incident study. *BMJ* **314**:870–874.

Armstrong D, Reyburn H and Jones R (1996) A study of general practitioners reasons for changing their prescribing behaviour. *BMJ* **312**:949–952.

Bandura A (1986) *Social Foundations of Thought and Action; A Social Cognitive Theory.* Englewood Cliffs, NJ: Prentice-Hall.

Baker R, Robertson N and Farooqi A (1995) Audit in general practice: factors influencing participation. *BMJ* **311**:31–34.

Barlow DH, Hayes SC and Nelson RO (1986) *The Scientist Practitioner: Research and Accountability in Clinical and Educational Settings*, Third Edition. New York: Pergamon.

Closs J and Cheater FM (1996) Audit or research – what is the difference? *J Clin Nurs* **5**:249–256.

Davis DA, Thomson MA, Oxman AD and Haynes RB (1995) Changing physician performance. A systematic review of the effect of continuing education strategies. *JAMA* **274**:700–705.

Fowkes FGR (1982) Medical audit cycle: a review of methods and research in clinical practice. *Medical Education* **16**:228–238.

Funk SG, Champagne MT, Wiese RA and Tornquist EM (1991) BARRIERS: The barriers to research utilization scale. *Applied Nursing Research* **4**:39–45.

Greco PJ and Eisenberg JM (1993) Changing physicians practices. *N Engl J Med* **329**:1271–1273.

Grol R (1992) Implementing guidelines in general practice care. *Quality in Health Care* **1**:184–191.

Grol R and Wensing M (1995) Implementation of quality assurance and medical audit: general practitioners perceived obstacles and requirements. *Br J Gen Pract* **45**:548–552.

Haines A (1996) The science of perpetual change. *Br J Gen Pract* **46**:115–119.

Haines A and Jones R (1994). Implementing findings of research. *BMJ* **308**:1488–1492.

Handy C (1993) *Understanding Organisations.* Fourth edition. London: Penguin.

Harrison (1972) How to describe your organization. *Harvard Business Review* Sept–Oct.

Janis IL (1972) *Victims of Groupthink.* Boston: Houghton Mifflin.

Kanouse DE and Jaccoby I (1988). When does information change practitioners behaviour? *Int J Technology Assessment in Health Care* **4**:27–33.

Lomas J (1994) Teaching old (and not so old) docs new tricks: effective ways to implement research findings. In: Dunn EV, Norton PG, Stewart M, Tudiver F and Bass MJ (editors) *Disseminating Research/Changing Practice.* Thousand Oaks: Sage Publications.

Manchester Open Learning (1993) *Planning and Managing Change.* London: Kogan Page.

Mazzuca SA (1986) The role of clinical environment in the translation of research into practice. *The Diabetes Educator* **12**:219–225.

Moscovici S (1985) Social influence and conformity. In: Lindzey G and Aronson E (editors) *Handbook of Social Psychology*, vol 2. New York: Random House, pp 115–150.

Oxman AD, Thomson MA, Davis DA and Haynes RB (1995) No magic bullets: systematic review of 102 trials of interventions to improve professional practice. *Can Med Assoc J* **153**:1423–1431.

Prochaska JO and DiClemente CC (1992) Stages of change in the modification of problem behaviours. In: Hersen M, Eisler RM and Miller PM (editors) *Progress in Behaviour Modification*. Sycamore, IL: Sycamore Press.

Prochaska JO, DiClemente CC and Norcross J (1992) In search of how people change. *Am Psychol* **47**:1102–1114.

Robertson N, Baker R and Hearnshaw H (1996) Changing the clinical behaviour of doctors: a psychological perspective. *Quality in Health Care* **5**:51–54.

Rogers E (1983) *Diffusion of Innovations*. New York: Free Press.

Stocking B (1992) Promoting change in clinical care. *Quality in Health Care* **1**:56–60.

Warr P (1996) *Psychology at Work*. Fourth edition. London: Penguin.

Worden JW (1987) *Grief Counselling and Grief Therapy*. Second edition. New York: Tavistock Publications.

Zajonc RB (1965) Social facilitation. *Science* **1429**:269–274.

Zimbardo PG and Leippe MR (1991) *The Psychology of Attitude Change and Social Influence*. Philadelphia: Temple University Press.

Chapter 4

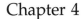

OVERCOMING OBSTACLES TO CHANGES

Hilary Hearnshaw and Richard Baker

People do not resist change, they resist being changed (Scholtes, 1988)

4.1 INTRODUCTION

Previous chapters have presented information from research studies of methods of implementing change, and discussed how theories of human behaviour can be used to guide the identification to obstacles to change and the choice of appropriate strategies to overcome them. Evidence and theories are essential, but how can they be put into practice? In this chapter, we discuss how this can be achieved. To illustrate the points, we will use the hypothetical case study introduced in Box 4.1.

4.2 THE TRADITIONAL METHOD OF IMPLEMENTING CHANGE IN AUDIT

There are good reasons for choosing to audit the use of thrombolytic treatment. There is good quality evidence that confirms that this treatment reduces mortality in patients who have a myocardial infarction, provided it is given soon after the onset of symptoms (Gershlick and More, 1998). The longer the delay, the less effective the treatment, and with a 24-h delay the benefits are limited. Despite the availability of convincing evidence, there have been delays in the adoption of thrombolysis in routine practice (Antman et al, 1992), and the proportion of patients who receive treatment varies between different hospitals. In one study of five hospitals, the proportions ranged from 39% to 89% (Robinson et al, 1996). The quality of the evidence, and the importance of reducing mortality in a common and frequently fatal condition might be thought sufficient to ensure that clinicians would generally administer

Implementing Change With Clinical Audit. Edited by Richard Baker, Hilary Hearnshaw and Noelle Robertson.
© 1999 John Wiley & Sons, Ltd.

Box 4.1   Case study – the first steps

Dr Judith Wilson was a consultant in accident and emergency medicine. She had read an article about the use of thrombolytic treatment in accident and emergency departments (Hood et al, 1998) and decided to undertake an audit. In the article, consultants in accident and emergency departments had been asked whether patients with heart attack (acute myocardial infarction) were routinely given thrombolysis in their department, and if not, whether this should be the case. Giving thrombolysis in the department rather than waiting for the patient to be admitted to a ward reduces the delay before treatment is started and hence can reduce mortality. The finding of the article was that although thrombolysis was given routinely in only 35% of departments, 58% of consultants thought they should. In Dr Wilson's department, there was no agreed policy on the routine use of thrombolysis.

Dr Wilson discussed the issue with colleagues, including her fellow consultants and senior nurses. They decided to check how many patients were given thrombolysis in the department, and to assess the delay before patients received treatment (sometimes referred to as door to needle time). They could then compare themselves to published information from studies in other departments (Nee et al, 1994). She asked the audit co-ordinator of the hospital for help in undertaking the audit. Data were collected over 12 weeks about all patients attending the department with suspected myocardial infarction. The criteria were:

1   In the absence of specific contraindications, the patient with strongly suspected acute myocardial infarction will receive thrombolytic therapy in the accident and emergency department.
2   The door to needle time will be 45 min or less.

The standards for both criteria were set at 80%.

thrombolytics, and that audit would be successful. What happened in our case study is shown in Box 4.2.

The methods chosen for implementing change in our hypothetical case study are typical of those used in many audits. The data were presented to some or all of the relevant clinicians, and a general agreement about the most appropriate clinical policy emerged from discussion. There are reasonable arguments to support this approach. For example, it may be supposed that by bringing the clinicians together in a group to discuss the results, the eventual policy will be more likely to be practical and have the commitment of all involved. Clinical care in an accident and emergency department relies on co-operation and team-work, and a group meeting to consider the audit findings is more likely to

---

Box 4.2   Case study – the first data collection

A meeting was arranged to review the results of the first data collection. The consultants, junior doctors, two invited cardiologists, and nursing staff attended, and the results were presented by the audit co-ordinator. They found that 32% of patients had received thrombolytics in the accident department. A further 40% received treatment after transfer from the department to the cardiac unit. For those receiving treatment in the department, only 42% met the criterion for door to needle time, and the mean delay was 62 min. For those treated in the cardiac unit, the delay was 146 min.

There was disappointment at the results. After some discussion, it was agreed that treatment should be commenced in the department whenever possible. The strategy chosen for distributing information about this policy, and for reminding staff in the department about it, was the posting of a note on the department notice board. The note was signed jointly by the heads of the departments of accident and emergency, and cardiology.

---

reflect, and build on, this normal pattern of work. If feedback had been limited to a written report sent to individuals, there may have been no opportunity to consider the report and arrive at a joint plan of action for improving care.

The plan for posting the new policy is also commonly used in audits, and it does have some arguments in its favour. It is unlikely that all relevant clinicians could have been present at the group meeting, and they need to be informed about the new policy. In addition, all staff are likely to need reminding of the policy. Reminders can be effective (see Chapter 1), and when they carry the authority of the heads of the departments concerned, they may be even more effective. Given these arguments, it is reasonable to anticipate that improvements in care will take place. However, as many involved in audit have come to realize, optimism about the prospects of change is often misplaced, as shown in the next stage of the case study (Box 4.3). In this example, the potential levers for change were unable to overcome the prevailing obstacles.

4.3   IDENTIFYING OBSTACLES – THE SYSTEMATIC APPROACH TO IMPLEMENTING CHANGE

4.3.1   Principles

It was explained in Chapter 1 that many methods have been tried for implementing change, some of which work some of the time. Chapter 2 considered how audit should be undertaken to provide objective evidence to guide the

Box 4.3   Case study – the second data collection

Six months later, the second data collection took place. Since the same types of patients were included, and the same methods were used, the data in the two collections were directly comparable. Once again, the co-ordinator reported the results to a meeting of those involved.

The proportion of patients receiving treatment in the department had risen from 32% to 37%, and 38% of these were within the door to needle time of 45 min. The mean delay had increased to 68 min. Calculation of confidence intervals indicated that the changes, such as they were, were most likely due to chance. The group was disappointed. Dr Judith Wilson wondered what had gone wrong.

need for change, and Chapter 3 suggested that implementation strategies should be chosen to match the particular obstacles to change that may be present. In this approach, the initial step is the identification of the prevailing obstacles. In the case study, this could have been undertaken either when the findings of the first data collection became available, or when the findings of the second data collection had shown that the first attempt to implement change had failed.

There are points in favour of identifying obstacles at either of these stages in the audit cycle. By identifying them early in the audit, the time and energy wasted in a futile attempt to implement change would be avoided. On the other hand, if the identification of obstacles is delayed until the second data collection has been completed, needless effort might be avoided – change may have occurred, making analysis of obstacles unnecessary. The decision about when to investigate obstacles rests on two factors. The first is the amount of effort needed to identify the obstacles. A detailed study of the obstacles may be difficult to justify in a setting that has already undertaken several audits and developed some understanding of the obstacles likely to be present locally. If a reasonable assessment can be made of which obstacles will be present, lengthy investigation would not be appropriate. However, if change fails to occur, the initial assessment of the obstacles is probably wrong and a more detailed investigation is then essential.

In the case study, both data collections demonstrated failure to achieve the standards that had been set. How might the obstacles to change be identified? To 'diagnose' them, we need to gather evidence from the beliefs, thoughts and behaviours of the people involved. The process of diagnosis involves the collection of information about 'symptoms' in people's own words and through observation of their behaviour and their systems of work, very much as a health professional would take a clinical history. A diagnosis can then be proposed on the basis of the symptoms, using progressive hypothesis testing as described in Chapter 3.

The following simple example illustrates how many of us use this approach in daily life. A young son switched to a new class at school is unlikely to volunteer information to his mother about his lack of self-esteem and fear of failure, or even information on his thoughts that he will not be able to keep up with his new classmates. He will probably say that he does not like it in the new class, does not like the new teacher, or that his classmates are unfriendly. His mother could, though, choose to ask questions that elicit more accurate and specific reasons. This method of simple questioning and listening is a normal social skill that many of us have and which can be applied to the task of identifying obstacles to change without too much difficulty.

Here are some examples of the questions an audit co-ordinator or interviewer could ask. 'How do you feel about this problem?' – this is a very open question that allows the respondent to set the agenda and talk about the things important to him or her. 'What would it be like if this change were implemented?' – this too is an open question, but the specific consideration of a possible change can focus people on the likely outcomes. This may provide an opportunity for obstacles to be identified from the negative consequences anticipated from the change. Other questions might be 'What obstacles might there be to this change?'; 'What would make it easier to do this?'; 'What would be the benefits of this change for you?'.

Here are some examples of responses that might lead to the diagnosis of the prevailing obstacles. The obstacle of low belief in personal ability (self-efficacy, see Chapter 3) could be indicated by phrases such as 'It would be very difficult for me to achieve that', or 'Some patients are very difficult to convince', or 'It has always been done by the physiotherapists, not the nurses, they are much better at it than we are'.

4.3.2 Guidance from research

A growing number of studies has investigated obstacles to change. DiCaccavo and Reid (1995) demonstrated that doctors are able to reflect on their own clinical behaviour and identify specific difficulties or obstacles they experience. This study investigated the pressure doctors feel in decision making and found that lack of time, dealing with uncertainty, and patient characteristics were the major issues. Berrow et al (1997) identified three obstacles to changing policies to comply with research evidence in three obstetric units – concerns about the adequacy or completeness of the evidence, concerns about the applicability of the evidence in the local setting, and concerns about local capabilities for acting on the evidence. These concerns reflected the clinical staff's justification for operating policies that conflicted with the evidence. After the study was completed, two of the units taking part changed their policies. The authors surmised that the staff of the units were given sufficient information during the study to enable the obstacles to be overcome. The latest, summarized research evidence had been made easily available and was endorsed by the Royal College of Obstetricians and Gynaecologists; the policy had been reviewed independently by the study team and the reasons for not applying the evidence could not be justified. Thus, almost by accident, the obstacles were removed and the changes were implemented.

The studies of DiCavacco and Reid (1995) and Berrow et al (1997) used interviews with staff to investigate obstacles. In other studies, marketing methods such as focus groups or surveys of targeted providers have been used to identify obstacles (Thomson et al, 1997). In this systematic review of 18 trials of educational outreach, marketing techniques were used in five trials, most of which were concerned with prescribing behaviour. For example, in a study of three types of medication, doctors typical of those included in the study were interviewed by a market research consultant to investigate their reasons for choosing these drugs (Avorn and Soumerai, 1983). In a second trial of prescribing psychoactive drugs for patients in nursing homes, nurses and doctors working in homes were interviewed to inform the preparation of educational materials to be used (Avorn et al, 1992). In marketing, focus groups are also commonly used to explore the views of typical potential customers. Although such methods of investigating obstacles may be relatively simple to use, they may still be too complex or take too much time for them to be routinely used in all audits. These studies serve to illustrate the potential for identifying obstacles, but approaches suitable for daily use are required.

4.3.3 Practical approaches

A questionnaire survey offers one approach. A disadvantage of questionnaires is that they limit the opportunity of respondents to express their views – there may be no questions on the topic of greatest importance to a particular respondent. There can be many different obstacles, and they can arise at the level of the organization or team as well as within individuals themselves. A questionnaire that does not consider all these possibilities may not be helpful.

Standard questionnaires can address some of these problems if they have been developed following investigation of the most common obstacles, and tested through repeated use. One example is the BARRIERS instrument devised in the USA for use with nurses (Funk et al, 1991). During the development of this instrument, existing literature and interviews with nurses were used to generate potential questions. These were pilot tested, and the eventual scale had 29 questions in four sub-scales: characteristics of the adopter, characteristics of the organization, characteristics of the innovation, and characteristics of the communication. Instruments such as this would appear to have considerable potential in guiding the choice of implementation strategies, but they have rarely been used. Also, the number of such instruments is limited, and on most occasions it will be necessary to devise a questionnaire *de novo*.

Although detailed interviews may require expertise and resources, simpler techniques can readily be applied. Brief, but structured, interviews may be all that is needed. Training for undertaking this type of interview is probably not needed. Notes should be taken during such interviews, and the analysis can be limited to a simple summary of the responses for feeding back to the group. A topic guide for use in our case study is shown in Table 4.1.

The methods suggested thus far have generally relied on asking individuals about the prevailing obstacles to change. Because obstacles can arise at the level of the health care team or group, it can also be helpful to ask groups of professionals about obstacles. Once again, practical methods are available. These generally rely on the groups concerned in the audit drawing on their own knowledge of the problems to identify those likely to be most important. The skills required are those of teamwork and the facilitation of the group. The use of brainstorming alone can generate a list of possible obstacles to change that the group can discuss and decide which are probably the most important. If the process of care is relatively complex, the group can develop a diagram of the care pathway or critical path (Joint Commission, 1994). This can often make clear the most likely source of problems. Further analysis can be undertaken by preparing a fishbone diagram and collecting data to indicate the most common obstacles (see Chapter 1).

The investigation of obstacles arising from the team itself may require the use of other methods. Observation alone may suggest that the influence of a powerful minority or groupthink is the cause of the problem. More detailed assessment of teamwork may consider factors such as the level of participation, whether there are shared objectives, and support for innovation (Tjosvold, 1991; Poulton and West, 1997). Problems of this type may demand a review of team leadership or the support of a skilled facilitator (see Chapter 7). Inferences about the obstacles acting at the level of the organization may be made from interviews with professionals. Additional information may be sought about the organizational structure, methods and speed of decision making, and orientation to short-term solutions rather than long-term goals (Williamson, 1992).

4.4 CHOOSING STRATEGIES

Having identified the prevailing obstacles to change, an appropriate implementation strategy must be selected. Several of the remaining chapters address this

Table 4.1   A topic guide for a brief, structured interview of the obstacles to change in the audit of thrombolytic therapy

1. Do you believe that the use of thrombolytics should be improved in the ways suggested?
2. Is this a widely held opinion in the department?
3. Why do you think we have failed to reach our target standards?
4. Are there any factors that are hindering you?
4. What would help us to reach the standards?

question. We will only outline the main points to consider here. It is important to point out that a detailed understanding of behavioural theories is not required, a simple but systematic approach can be adopted on most occasions.

On reviewing the information about obstacles to change, a practical solution may be obvious immediately. Some obstacles to change may be caused by the lack of a simple piece of equipment, an agreed policy or a revised system of work. In these circumstances, the strategy is straightforward, and consists of resolving the deficiency. Sometimes, the obstacle is insurmountable. For example, if the only solution would be building a new hospital, or appointing large numbers of new staff, those undertaking the audit will be unable to take any effective action. The best approach in these circumstances would be to admit defeat and consider audit of another topic. However, it would be important to ensure the findings are communicated to managers and policy makers, who would then be able to address the problem when developing long-term plans. After all, new hospitals are built from time to time.

On most occasions, obstacles to change are neither immediately soluble nor totally impossible to resolve. With a little thought, potentially successful strategies can usually be identified. This process is assisted by awareness of the variety of strategies that are available, and some past experience of using one or two of them. Furthermore, by making sure that the obstacles and the circumstances of the people who face them are fully understood, the most appropriate strategy will often emerge. The case study shows how this can occur. Two hypothetical scenarios are shown, each dealing with different obstacles (Boxes 4.4 and 4.5). Different methods were used to identify the obstacles, and different strategies were chosen. The process in each case relied on careful observation of individuals or groups, and the targeted application of common sense.

Professionals who frequently have responsibility for audits should be able to assess obstacles to change and select strategies more systematically than the approach illustrated in the case study. They should become familiar with one or two theories of behaviour change (discussed in Chapter 3), although a detailed knowledge of all theories is not needed. It is also important to develop an understanding of the obstacles that can arise in health care teams or groups of professionals (see Chapter 7). Similarly, familiarity with a variety of strate-

Box 4.4 Implementing change – scenario one

Dr Wilson discussed the disappointing results with several members of the accident and emergency department staff. She talked with the staff individually, and asked them for their views on the reasons why there had been little improvement. The main factor that emerged from these discussions was the attitude of a highly respected consultant in the department. This colleague of Dr Wilson accepted that thrombolysis was an effective treatment, but was uncertain about its safety when given in a hurry in the department. When thrombolysis was first being introduced, two patients he treated had died, one from a subarachnoid haemorrhage and the other had a missed diagnosis of dissecting aortic aneurysm. Because he was so respected, the views of this consultant had a powerful influence on other members of the department, and many felt that thrombolysis was safer when delayed until patients could be fully assessed in the cardiac unit.

Instead of confronting her colleague directly, which may have reinforced his reluctance to change, Dr Wilson thought it would be more effective to present him with evidence about the safety of early administration of thrombolysis in a setting which would allow him, and other members of the department, to consider the issue in detail and reach their own conclusions. She decided to invite a consultant from the accident department of a nearby hospital who was widely recognized as an expert on the topic. She arranged a seminar, made sure that her colleague was attending, and invited all members of the department. The invited speaker was asked to address the issue of the safety of thrombolytics, and he was able to draw on data that he had collected in his own department. Dr Wilson facilitated the discussion, ensuring that those present acknowledged the anxieties about early treatment, but accepted that new information reported by the invited expert now showed that early treatment was preferable to delay.

After the meeting, Dr Wilson noted that members of the department expressed more positive views about early treatment, and a third data collection 6 months later showed that the proportion of patients receiving early treatment had increased to 62%, and the door to needle time had fallen to 40 min.

gies is needed (see Chapter 1). When this level of knowledge is unable to resolve the obstacles to change in an audit, it is time to seek advice from a specialist. Psychologists may have useful suggestions, and since many hospitals have psychologists as members of staff, they may be locally accessible. There are many other behavioural and organizational experts, although their advice may be expensive. However, it is likely that in most audits the change process can be helped to succeed by using the systematic approach to identifying and overcoming obstacles, described here.

Box 4.5   Implementing change – scenario two

After some thought, Dr Wilson asked the audit co-ordinator for advice about investigating the reasons for lack of improvement. The co-ordinator suggested brief interviews of members of the department, and she interviewed selected junior and senior medical and nursing staff. The findings indicated problems in communication in the department. Decisions were usually made by one or two senior staff, the others being expected to act as instructed. Communication in the opposite direction, from junior to senior staff, was limited, and in consequence the senior staff were unable to understand all the practical implications of their instructions. In particular, they were unaware of the problems caused by department policies on the storage of thrombolytic medication, rules for its administration, and the pressures to complete patients' initial assessment and admission procedures as quickly as possible.

Dr Wilson discussed these findings with a friend who was a manager in industry, and discovered that problems of this type were a common cause of poor implementation by teams. Together with the co-ordinator, she convened a meeting of members of the department. They used brainstorming to identify all the problems staff faced in using thrombolytic medication, and helped the group draw a fishbone diagram to assist in analysing the principal, practical obstacles. Throughout, Dr Wilson made sure that all members of the group took part in the discussions, and controlled the input of senior staff. As a result, a new system for supervising thrombolytic treatment was introduced, which reduced some of the organizational obstacles. Six months later, the third data collection showed that improvements had finally been achieved.

4.5 SUMMARY POINTS

- Obstacles may be identified before attempting to implement change, or when the second data collection has shown that change has not taken place.
- There are practical methods for identifying obstacles, including brief interviews, questionnaires, observation, and group meetings.
- Often, the selection of a strategy to overcome obstacles is straightforward once the obstacles have been identified. A detailed knowledge of behavioural theories is not needed.
- Those who undertake audit frequently should become familiar with a few theories of behaviour change, and with the range of implementation strategies available.
- When the obstacles are more complex, or change continues to be elusive, it may help to call on the advice of an expert on behaviour change such as a psychologist.

- Sometimes, the obstacle to change is insurmountable. It is then best to inform management and move on to an alternative topic for audit.

REFERENCES

Antman EM, Lau J, Kupelnick B, Mosteller F and Chalmers TC (1992) A comparison of results of meta-analyses of randomised controlled trials and recommendations of experts. *JAMA* **268**:240–248.

Avorn J and Soumerai SB (1983) Improving drug-therapy decisions through educational outreach. A randomized controlled trial of academically based 'detailing'. *N Engl J Med* **308**:1457–1463.

Avorn J, Soumerai SB, Everitt DE, Ross-Degnan D, Beers MH, Sherman D, Salam-Schatz SR and Fields D (1992) A randomized trial of a program to reduce the use of psychoactive drugs in nursing homes. *N Engl J Med* **327**:168–173.

Berrow D, Humphrey C and Hayward J (1997) Understanding the relation between research and clinical policy: a study of clinicians' views. *Quality in Health Care* **6**:181–186.

DiCaccavo A and Reid F (1995). Decisional conflict in general practice: strategies of patient management. *Soc Sci Med* **41**:347–353.

Funk SG, Champagne MT, Wiese RA and Tornquist EM (1991). BARRIERS: the barriers to research utilisation scale. *Applied Nursing Research* **4**:39–45.

Gershlick AH and More RS (1998) Treatment of myocardial infarction. *BMJ* **316**:280–284.

Hood S, Birnie D, Swan L and Hillis WS (1998) Questionnaire survey of thrombolytic treatment in accident and emergency departments in the United Kingdom. *BMJ* **316**:274.

Joint Commission on Accreditation of Healthcare Organisations (1994) *Forms, Charts & Other Tools for Performance Improvement*. Illinois: JCAHO.

Nee PA, Gray AJ and Martin MA (1994) Audit of thrombolysis initiated in an accident and emergency department. *Quality in Health Care* **3**:29–33.

Poulton B and West M (1997) Defining and measuring effectiveness for primary health care teams. In: Pearson P and Spencer J (eds) *Promoting Teamwork in Primary Care*. London: Arnold.

Robinson MB, Thompson E and Black NA (1996) Evaluation of the effectiveness of guidelines, audit and feedback: improving the use of intravenous thrombolysis in patients with suspected acute myocardial infarction. *International Journal for Quality in Health Care* **8**:211–222.

Scholtes PR (1988) *The Team Handbook: How to Improve Quality with Teams*. Madison, WI: Joiner Associates.

Thomson MA, Oxman AD, Davis DA, Haynes RB, Freemantle N and Harvey EL (1997) Outreach visits to improve health professional practice and health care outcomes. In: Bero L, Grilli R, Grimshaw J and Oxman A (eds) Collaboration on Effective Professional Practice Module of *The Cochrane Database of Systematic Reviews* (updated 1 September 1997). Available in the Cochrane Library. The Cochrane Collaboration; issue 4. Oxford: Update Software.

Tjosvold D (1991) *Team Organization. An Enduring Competitive Advantage*. Chichester: John Wiley & Sons.

Williamson P (1992) From dissemination to use: management and organisational barriers to the application of health services research findings. *Health Bull* **50**:78–86.

Chapter 5

AUDIT AND LEARNING

George Brown, Gifford Batstone and Mary Edwards

In this chapter, we explore the subtle relationships between audit and learning. The purpose of the chapter is to demonstrate how an understanding of the processes of audit can enhance the learning process and, *vice versa*, how an understanding of the processes of learning can enhance the audit process. We begin with the process of audit and the audit cycle. This naturally leads to a consideration of various perspectives on learning and their relationships with audit and the audit cycle. Throughout the chapter, practical suggestions for conducting audit are provided.

5.1 AUDIT IS A FORM OF ASSESSMENT

A detailed account of audit as an iterative process has been provided in Chapter 1. Here we wish to remind readers that audit is part of the *genus* of assessment. Audit is essentially concerned with matching existing procedures against desirable standards, with a view to improving procedures. Its near relatives are appraisal, total quality management, quality assessment, quality assurance and quality control. More distant relatives are performance review, competency-based assessment and the assessment of student learning.

Given that audit is a form of assessment, it is hardly surprising that, like student assessment, it has intimate links with learning and it contains inherent conflicts. Like all forms of assessment, audit influences the nature of learning and performance. Just as changing the mode of assessment changes the mode of student learning, so too does auditing the performance of a clinical team, on given criteria, change performance towards those criteria. If the criteria are not appropriate for the purposes of the task then the team may end up fulfilling the criteria but not performing the task well.

Implementing Change With Clinical Audit. Edited by Richard Baker, Hilary Hearnshaw and Noelle Robertson.
© 1999 John Wiley & Sons, Ltd.

All forms of assessment, including audit, are based upon the common procedures of taking a sample, drawing inferences and estimating worth. Common
weaknesses are:

- The sample does not match the stated outcomes.
- The sample is drawn from too narrow a domain.
- The sample is too large or too small.
- Absence of well defined standards.
- Unduly specific criteria.
- Variations in the inferences drawn by different auditors or assessors of the
  sample.
- Variations in estimates of worth.

The content of the sample in audit may be, for example, patient records, referrals, emergency treatment and doctor/patient communication skills. The
method of sampling may be an analysis of records, direct observations, questionnaires, interviews and discussions. The clinical audit itself may be undertaken by oneself, a clinical team, other peers or, increasingly, by patients. The
process of making inference may involve quantitative measures and/or qualitative descriptions. The estimates of worth may be based upon norms, ideals or
achievable standards. Lurking beneath this description of the processes of audit
are deep questions of values and purposes.

The primary purpose of audit is to estimate the worth of activities. Once this
worth has been established, other purposes come into play. In assessment in
general, the most notable are: the licence to proceed, rank ordering and the
provision of feedback. The first two are related to criterion-referenced assessment and normative assessment. Audit may be primarily *formative*, that is, it
may provide feedback that assists a clinical team to reflect upon its goals and on
ways of improving. Alternatively, it may be primarily *summative*, providing a
series of judgements or recommendations. In practice, the distinction between
formative and summative assessment is not clear cut. Summative assessment
can, if expressed appropriately, provide meaningful and useful feedback and
thereby aid development. Formative feedback may involve multiple points of
summative feedback. Both summative and formative audit (and assessment)
involve judgements. There are conflicts between the judgemental and developmental purposes of audit. Achieving a satisfactory balance that pleases all those
concerned is not easy. Figure 5.1 provides a simple model for exploring the
relationships between these aspects of audit.

The continuum in Figure 5.1 is not a pure diagonal. Judgemental audit has
developmental effects and judgements need to be made to enable improvements to occur. However, difficulties arise if judgemental and developmental
purposes are competing. A practice, clinical team or an individual clinician may
be willing to improve, but unwilling to reveal inadequacies. Neither private
companies nor individuals are usually willing to reveal evidence that could be

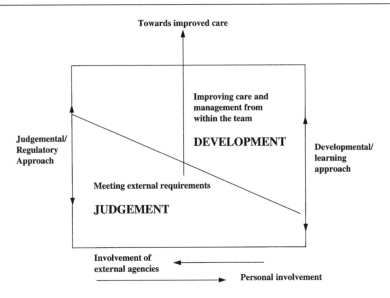

Figure 5.1 Judgement and development in audit

used against them by their competitors or managers. For these reasons, it is suggested that formative and summative audit are separated. Formative audit should be used to provide constructive, confidential feedback to a clinical team. It might be undertaken by the team itself with a little help from 'critical friends'. Summative audit should be used to provide evaluations of past achievements that are open to public scrutiny. Different strategies and procedures are required for these types of audit, but both require sensitive handling.

There is, inevitably, debate about what counts as good assessment or audit. Issues of fairness, reliability, validity and feasibility predominate. Fairness implies equality of opportunity and treatment of the individuals or teams being audited. Reliability implies consistency of approach and validity implies appropriateness of methods of truth seeking. Feasibility raises the question of staff and material resources available, what is acceptable to clinical staff, what is practicable within resource constraints and the opportunity costs of audit. If the time and effort of audit exceed the value of the recommended changes, then audit may not be worthwhile. All of these are deep problems. Clearly, purposes and contexts are central to the debate on what counts as a good audit. Most people agree that:

- The purposes, dimensions and criteria should be clear to the auditors and the audited.
- They should be used consistently by the auditors.

- The sample of activities observed should be representative of the major dimensions being audited.
- The dimensions should be related to the purposes of the audit.
- The inferences drawn should be consistent.
- The estimates of worth should be consistent with the inferences and the criteria.

There remains a problem for a health care system. If it is to improve then monitoring, including audit, is necessary. However, if that monitoring is seen as threatening to the people involved, they will be reluctant to reveal information. One way of resolving the dilemma is to ensure that every clinical team has its own quality assurance system in place. If such an approach is used, the external agencies can be provided with evidence that such a system is in place, but not the detailed data generated by the system of audit. However, the external agencies may of course also receive data that are necessary for their systemic development, in particular, for their provision of hospital and community care, the pharmaceutical budget, building budgets and strategic planning and development.

5.2   SPECIFIC CHARACTERISTICS OF AUDIT

Clinical audit itself has been variously defined (see Chapter 1). For example, Marinker (1990, p. 7) defined audit as 'the attempt to improve the quality of medical care by measuring the performance of those that practise that care, by considering their performance in relation to desired standards, and by improving on this performance'. His definition raises questions about the nature of standards and whether it is always possible to improve upon existing performance. SCOPME (1989), rather than attempting a precise definition, offered the following characteristics of audit:

- Peer review: clinical audit is usually clinician led and conducted.
- Involves the setting of standards.
- Involves reviewing practice against these standards and assessing reasons for conformance or non-conformance directed at the quality of care.
- Requires the corporate commitment of the clinical team.
- Leads to change provided that the remedial action is taken which enhances the quality of care.

5.3   THE AUDIT CYCLE

Figure 5.2 provides a summary of the iterative process of the audit cycle. Each of these phases of the cycle has implications for learning – and issues of some complexity.

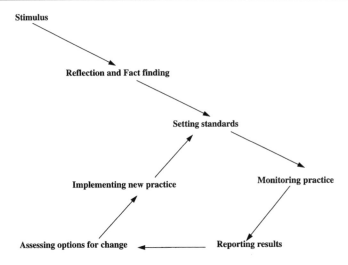

Figure 5.2   The audit cycle

Reflection and fact finding may involve the development of new modes of learning and investigation. Reflection is a process that has to be learnt. Fact finding involves literature searches and summarizing the relevant information.

The setting of standards presents difficulties for a system, the clinical team and an individual. A recent report suggests that this aspect of audit together with literature searches are a major weakness amongst general practitioner trainers and registrars (Lough and Murray, 1997). Informal discussions suggest that hospital-based doctors and other hospital staff experience similar difficulties. Often standards are based upon the most common practice, rather than upon an ideal or a set of explicit criteria based on evidence. What all do is not necessarily correct: it may be simply expedient. In the early stages of developing audit, it is often better to begin with the question: *what counts as good practice?* (in record keeping, care of elderly patients, consultative skills etc.) rather than with the question: *what standards should we adopt?* The use of guidelines and systematic reviews of literature are increasingly the source of criteria and standards as we move towards the enhancement of clinical care.

The monitoring of practice implies that there are criteria and methods of data collection. In the past, criteria have been implicit. The view of another professional or group of professionals was deemed sufficient even though the basis of their judgements may have been shrouded in mystery. The new drive towards openness requires the use of explicit criteria so that everyone may be clear what judgements are being made and on what basis. However, one should be wary of providing over detailed criteria for these may be ignored by users because they are too time-consuming (Mitchell and Cuthbert, 1989). Further, explicit criteria are not necessarily linked to only one standard. The same explicit criterion may fit more than one standard, and explicit criteria may lead to agreed standards rather than vice versa. The methods of data collection include the design of questionnaires, the use of focus groups, structured and in-depth interviews, various methods of direct observation and the use of quantitative and qualitative methods of analysis.

The report of an audit based on review findings requires careful consideration of how one communicates the findings as well as what one communicates. Aggressive confrontation is likely to lead to denial and hostility. Reports by an audit facilitator are likely to be dismissed, or the facilitator attacked verbally, by some senior managers or clinicians. If bad news is to be broken, then one should send early warning signals in the presentation and, perhaps, before the presentation. If persuasion is a key task then one would be wise to apply the principles given in Box 5.1.

Assessment of the options for change implies a need to explore the relevant literature and to examine critically the strengths and weaknesses of the options in relation to the context in which the clinical team is working. This, in itself, is a form of reflective learning.

Implementing new practice involves planning, learning, the collection of feedback and reflection.

It can be seen that the whole of the audit cycle is shot through with learning. The question then arises: what kinds of learning?

5.4   PERSPECTIVES ON LEARNING

To a novice, learning is about the absorption and regurgitation of facts. After all, many clinicians initially learnt anatomy in that way. However, as we grow in experience, we recognize that there are many different types of learning and many perspectives on learning. In the case study of an audit, reported in a subsequent section of this chapter, we outline some of the different types of learning. Here we are concerned with the major perspectives on learning: behaviourism, cognitive theory, experiential theory, humanistic theories, and their implications for the process of audit.

Behaviourism has its roots in the organization of industrial work for the masses. It values observable outcomes and objectives. It eschews introspection, thinking, feelings and self direction. In so doing it rejects a substantial part of human learning – and the inner reflective processes involved in audit. Not surprisingly, a behaviourist perspective appeals to health managers, for it emphasizes objectives, outcomes, competencies, targets and goals. Indeed, the most popular definition of learning has particular appeal: 'learning is the mod-

---

Box 5.1   Some pointers to persuasion

1. Know your participants and think what kinds of arguments may be appealing to them.
2. People are more likely to listen to you and accept your suggestions if you are already perceived as credible, trustworthy and having expertise.
3. When there are arguments for and against a procedure, it is usually better to present both sides.
4. If you have to stress risks in a procedure, do not overdo the arousal of fear.
5. Say what experts or expert groups do when faced with the problem you are discussing.
6. If the problem is complex for the group, you should draw the conclusion or at least give them time for discussion. If it is not too complex, let the group members draw their own conclusions.
7. If the suggestions you are making are likely to be challenged by others, describe their views in anticipation and show how they may be wrong.
8. If the task you are asking a group to do is complex, acknowledge that there is a risk of failure and the need for revision and reconsideration. Never say a new task is easy, rather say it may not be easy at first.
9. If a task is threatening admit it is and consider ways of reducing that threat.
10. Do not deride cherished traditions. Instead, show how the approach links to those traditions or indicate that people used to hold that view but that it is no longer appropriate.
11. Do not deride people for their views. Instead state that their views were correct but the changes in the context and of knowledge suggest a new approach is required.

(From Brown et al, 1997)

---

ification of observable behaviour' (Hilgard, 1962). The definition of 'observable' is problematic. Observable how and when? Often one has to infer change from observable behaviours. Further, there may be no immediately observable change in behaviour. Improvement in health as a result of improvement in audit, health assurance or continuing professional development may not be observable for some years.

The criticisms of naive behaviourism led subsequently to another definition of learning. Learning is conceived as: 'the changes in knowledge, skills, understanding and attitudes brought about by experience and reflection' (Brown et al, 1997). This definition encompasses much of the work on cognitive learning (Ausubel, 1989), student learning (Entwistle, 1992), experiential learning (Kolb,

1984; Boud et al, 1985) and reflective learning (Kolb, 1984; Boud et al, 1985; Schon, 1983, 1988).

More recently, the notion of learning as the construction of meaning has re-emerged. This constructivism is based on the notion that people construct personal meanings and theories about their world. The approach emphasizes the individual nature of learning. It is related to the work of Piaget and Inhelder (1969) and Vygotsky (1962) on development and notions of post-modernism. Finally, there are perspectives that are concerned with personal growth and maturation, and in particular, with how changes in inner states change the way people perceive and respond to their worlds (Rogers, 1969, 1983; Maslow, 1973; Roth, 1990).

All of these perspectives are relevant to audit but each has limitations as well as strengths.

5.5   THE USE OF BEHAVIOURISTIC PRINCIPLES

Standards, explicit criteria and behavioural objectives are part of the repertoire of behaviourism and they provide a clear framework for action. The use of standards and explicit criteria is a *sine qua non* for an audit. One needs standards and criteria to enable judgements to be made.

There are pitfalls, however, in the use of criteria and standards. First, too detailed a set of criteria can be overwhelming. For example, few hospital staff would willingly complete a five-page checklist on the performance of a junior nurse or house officer on a relatively minor task. Most people resort to making a global judgement and then filling in the criteria quickly (Mitchell and Cuthbert, 1989). Criteria need to be explicit but sufficiently broad to ensure that they are used effectively. Second, the focus upon standards can result in the reporting of actions rather than focusing upon *informed* actions. A third relative danger is short-termism. People fill in an audit form and then forget it until the next time. The more remote the source of the audit form, the greater the likelihood of the form being ignored in practice. Check-lists are particularly prone to this danger. A list of standards and competencies is no guarantee of quality care. Fourthly, a danger is that, paradoxically, detailed criteria may promote over-dependence. Put rather crudely, the message to a clinical team is 'if you do X, Y and Z you will be regarded as successful'. That form of success reinforces conformity and dependence rather than encouraging creativity, the development of new approaches and the development of an independent professional judgement. Finally, standards and their related criteria are *indicators* of performance. They do not provide clear guidelines for learning, indeed, they can reduce audit to the learning of audit indicators and the immediately relevant bits of knowledge. Fragmentation, short termism and over dependence then are serious risks. The processes of audit necessarily involve other notions: the notions of active, flexible, reflective learning.

5.6   HOW DO PEOPLE LEARN?

Most people learn best when they are active, the learning task is perceived as relevant, the learning environment is safe, the objectives of learning are clear and the perceived needs are satisfied. These principles are derived from studies of student learning (Entwistle, 1987), the work of adult educators (Brookfield, 1986; Knowles, 1990) and studies of change management (Beckard and Pritchard, 1992; Pettigrew et al, 1992; Handy, 1993).

Entwistle's research on styles of learning indicates that there are two predominant styles: knowledge-seeking and understanding-seeking (see Box 5.2). Knowledge-seeking is essentially concerned with information search and retrieval, whereas understanding-seeking is predominantly concerned with the search for meaning and the deeper concepts and processes involved. A pathology commonly associated with knowledge-seeking is the reluctance to take decisions on the basis of evidence collected. Consequently, more and more evidence is collected and never used to take decisions. A common pathology

---

Box 5.2   Orientations to learning

Knowledge seeker
Aims to store facts, or concepts.
Collects skills, procedures.
Breaks down problems and tasks into separate sub-units.
Makes links within units of knowledge.
Uses memorization skills.
Works methodically through logical order of task problems.
Analyses.
Uses systematic trial and error.

Understanding seeker
Tries to relate information or task to own experience.
Makes links to other bodies or knowledge.
Restructures for personal meaning.
Synthesizes.
Likes to work from 'whole' picture.
Searches for underlying structure, purpose, and meaning.
Intuitive use of evidence.
Uses analogies, metaphors.

of understanding-seeking is to 'globe trot', to over-generalize on the basis of insufficient evidence. Both knowledge-seeking and understanding-seeking are necessary for the development of critical thinking and, therefore, important for all the phases of the audit cycle. The two pathologies of learning are also inherent dangers in the processes of audit.

Brookfield (1986) suggests that the key principles underlying self-directed learning are:

- Voluntary participation.
- Mutual respect of other professionals and their roles.
- Collaborative spirit in seeking a common goal.
- Practice – a set of examples to be practised to promote and implement change.
- Critical reflection on current practice.
- Self direction.

These principles are relevant to the conditions of learning as well as to the motivation to learn. Work on the management of change (see Brown et al, 1997) indicates that for the probability of change to be maximized the following conditions are necessary:

- Participants in the audit recognize the problem as a problem for them.
- They are involved in developing a solution.
- There is a trial period.
- The solution is then reviewed.

These principles are in line with Power (1994), who argues that for audit to be effective, it must be local. The more remote the source of the audit from the group undertaking the audit, the less likely will the audit be internalized and accepted. Clearly this is a potential weakness of national and college audits. All of the above principles are relevant to all phases of the audit cycle and to the process of audit itself. A particular risk to audit, as a vehicle of learning and change, is the use of rigid, national standardized procedures. Such procedures may well provide face reliability and face validity but may not provide genuine reliability, validity and commitment.

5.7 THE IMPORTANCE OF REFLECTION IN LEARNING

Reflective learning is a key factor in helping a novice to develop into an expert (Schmidt et al, 1990). It led Schon (1988) to argue that professionals must learn how to frame and re-frame the complex and ambiguous problems they are facing and then interpret and modify their practice as a result. He distinguishes *reflection in action*, which is akin to immediate decision taking, and *reflection on action* that provides a longer and perhaps a deeper view. Both Boud et al (1995) and Cowan (1998) extend the notion of reflection to include *reflection for action*. These conceptions of reflective learning are at the heart of the audit process.

However, Hatton and Smith (1995) suggested that some precautions are necessary in the use of reflective learning. They point to the dangers of encouraging people to reflect too early in a task, at an inappropriate level and on too broad a topic. Their comments are apposite to the processes of audit. They also argue that reflective learning itself has to be learnt. They distinguish five types of reflective learning, in ascending order of complexity. These are:

- *Descriptive writing*, in which no reflection is evident.
- *Descriptive reflection*, in which some reasons, based on personal judgements, are provided.
- *Dialogic reflection*, in which a person explores possible reasons and approaches which are rooted in their reading of the relevant literature and their discussions with other professional colleagues.
- *Critical reflection*, that involved the exploration of reasons and approaches and the underlying assumptions and concepts. The exploration is based upon an evaluation of context as well as of the problem. It takes account of social, personal and organizational influences as well as the relevant literature.

The higher levels of reflection are, they indicate, augmented by discussion and feedback.

Perhaps the most relevant theory concerned with reflection was developed by Kolb (1976, 1984) and subsequently developed by Honey and Mumford (1983). Kolb identified four learning styles:

- *Activists* seem to learn most from short, here and now, activities and least from those that require a passive role.
- *Reflectors* do not like to be rushed. They prefer to learn through assimilating information, reflecting upon it and their experience, and reaching decisions in their own time.
- *Theorists* prefer to integrate observations and experience into a theoretical framework. They dislike situations and tasks in which they do not have the opportunity to explore in depth.
- *Pragmatists* seem to learn best from activities when they can see the practical value of the subject matter and when they can test ideas and techniques in practice. They dislike learning that seems unrelated to an immediately recognizable benefit or need.

People vary in their pre-dispositions towards these different learning styles. Very few people are totally locked into one style and very few are good at all four styles. In practice, they are probably influenced by context and purpose.

A reflector may become an activist as a deadline approaches. An activist may become a theorist if the task is framed appropriately.

Kolb suggests that the total learning cycle consists of observe practice, reflect, determine principles and standards (theorize), try out a new situation (experiment), observe practice. Figure 5.3 sets out the cycle. It bears a remarkable resemblance to the audit cycle.

Kolb's avowed concern is the process of learning, not the outcome. However, processes and outcomes are not that easily separated. An outcome may be an end point which becomes a new starting point. Thus learning is helical rather than cyclical. As a framework for learning, Kolb's theory has much to offer. However, there is a danger in assuming that the styles of learning are genetically fixed. Kolb's theory provides a useful input into the assessment of prior learning (Boud et al, 1985) and into self and peer assessment and feedback (Falchikov and Boud, 1989; Falchikov, 1996). These, together with the use of learning portfolios (Brown et al, 1997) and audit projects are valuable methods of learning. For audit, one also needs a light structural framework of standards in order to help clinical teams to match their perceptions against those of others. In particular, the notion of self-assessment needs much more attention. It can be notoriously inaccurate, if only because people wish to present themselves in a good light and to mask any deficiencies. It is a considerable challenge in audit to provide a context in which self-assessment can become more accurate and realistic, and self-development can lead to mature, informed judgement and action.

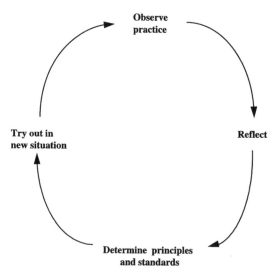

Figure 5.3 The learning cycle (based on Kolb, 1996)

5.8 PERSONAL GROWTH

As well as developing practical and cognitive skills, clinical audit and associated activities are concerned with personal development, with such features as self-confidence, self-esteem, initiative and understanding of oneself and others. Here the theories of personal growth become salient. Exponents of personal growth theories stress autonomy, trust, consultation, negotiation and reflection upon experience (Roth, 1990). Above all, they stress the importance of providing choice and responsibility for learning (Wittrock, 1986; Stevens, 1990). However, whilst there is evidence that freedom to learn is essential for intellectual development, there is also evidence that too much freedom does not actually help a person to develop, but rather brings about acute anxiety and distress (Stevens, 1990). In short, personal growth and freedom to learn need to be provided within a structured framework.

The focus of growth theories upon changing a person, his or her attitudes, perceptions and feelings, has other dangers. Attempts to change people rather than their situation might, unwittingly, be encouraging people to accept the status quo as good and mal-adaptation to it to be a form of personal or group failure. It may be as important to try to change one's world or even a health care system as to accept it. There is also an assumption amongst the advocates of personal growth that it is the deeper layers of feeling that shape human thought and actions. However, it is also likely that actions and cognitions can shape feelings and motivation (Brewin, 1988). Interaction within the individual as well as an interaction of the individual and his/her environment can shape and develop that person's learning, thinking and motivation.

This view of inner interaction is in line with the work of Heath (1964) and Perry (1981), who built on Heath's work. Heath describes the ideal student as 'the reasonable adventurer'. Perry goes on to suggest that learning is much more than the accumulation of facts, fine tuning and cognitive restructuring that is advocated by some cognitive psychologists (e.g. Norman, 1980). It is concerned with changes in feeling and attitudes towards others and towards oneself. It often involves the restructuring of one's commitment and priorities. This view is not limited to learning by medical and nursing undergraduates. When faced with new contexts or challenges, older clinicians can retreat into stereotyped primitive dualism and associated modes of behaviour. Hence the importance of laying the foundations of effective lifelong learning early in the undergraduate years of all health professionals.

Perry's stages of development are given in Box 5.3. It is likely that people who are fundamentalist in outlook or wedded strongly to extreme ideologies may have difficulty in going beyond stage one in Perry's scheme and therefore find troublesome the whole business of audit and the audit cycle.

Box 5.3   Perry's stages of development orientations to learning

Levels of intellectual and ethical development
1.   Learner seeks and expects right answers for everything.
2.   Learner perceives diversity as distraction.
3.   Learner accepts diversity as temporary.
4.   Diversity accepted but therefore 'everyone has a right to know'.
5.   Learner perceives all knowledge as contextual and relative.
6.   Learner perceives necessity of making a personal judgement as opposed to simple belief.
7.   Learner makes such a judgement and personal commitment.
8.   Learner explores implications of commitment.
9.   Learner experiences issues of personal identity in undertaking commitment.

(Based on Perry, 1981)

5.9   LINKS BETWEEN AUDIT, LEARNING AND EDUCATION

In describing the nature of audit and learning, we have shown the links between audit, as a species of assessment, and learning, and we have demonstrated that various perspectives on learning contribute to the audit process and the audit cycle. Indeed, these links are so strong that it might be argued that audit *is* a mode of learning.

This view of audit eventually permeated the thinking of the Department of Health (1994) in its document *The Evolution of Clinical Audit*. Prior to this, it considered audit primarily as an operational tool. It took the combined forces of the Royal College of Physicians (1989) and the Royal College of Surgeons (1989) to correct this perception. Even then, audit was seen as 'essentially educational' rather than as a learning process. Kenneth Clarke, when Secretary of State for Health, put it thus: 'Medical audit is about quality assurance in clinical work. As it entails a measurement of performance it must be a key part of continuing professional development.' (Clarke, 1990)

This point may seem casuistic, but there are important differences between formal education and learning. Learning requires only a task and a learner, or a set of learners. Formal education requires a teacher, a student or students, and a curriculum. The major differences between learning and formal education are given in Table 5.1. To these one might add a cautionary note that the set of items are, in effect, dimensions that carry spectra of possibilities. Some audits have the characteristics normally associated with formal education and vice

Table 5.1   Approaches to formal learning and audit

Traditional	Audit
Curriculum based	Needs based
Authoritarian	Rational
Teacher centred	Learner centred
Individual	Group
Competitive	Open
Accepting	Critical
Theoretical	Experiential

versa. Similarly, there are differences between continuing medical education and continuing professional development. Continuing education is a narrow concept which is based largely on lectures, seminars, courses and conferences outside of the work place. The term continuing professional development is now used more widely. It encompasses continuing education but it also includes:

- Acquisition/application of new knowledge in the clinical setting.
- Better application of existing knowledge in the clinical setting.
- Enhanced management of healthcare:
    working in clinical teams.
    working within the organization.
- Enhanced communication:
    with patients.
    within and between clinical teams.
    with managers.
- Improved learning skills.
- Improved assessment skills.
- Improved teaching skills.
- Attention to social, cultural, ethical and psychological influences in the work-place.
- Effective use of information technology.
- The process of maturation.

Continuing professional development emphasizes the importance of work-based and work-place learning, and of the use of methods of learning and assessment that can be used in work settings. This is not only because work place learning is less expensive, because of less loss of staff time, but primarily because it is probably a more effective way of bringing together research findings and practice, improving professional practice and promoting team development.

5.10 LINKS BETWEEN THE LEARNING AND AUDIT CYCLES

Figure 5.4 shows the major links between the learning cycle and the audit cycle. As one can see, the process of clinical audit involves the review of current processes against standards of care developed by team consensus. It is essentially a reflective learning process based primarily upon clinical experience. Consequently, in our discussion of the links between audit and learning we use the notions of learning *in* audit, learning *on* audit and learning *for* audit.

As indicated earlier, a major difficulty of the audit cycle is the setting of standards. For many, this is best achieved by observing practice and reflecting on its aims. This process is often triggered by an unexpected finding (for example, inadequate performance indicators, poor performance, adverse experience or complications of clinical treatment). It is often developed because of a desire for change. Once the aims of the observed practice have been determined, the setting of standards seems much simpler. The learning cycle may be triggered by the audit cycle or *vice versa*. The challenge in the learning cycle is the development of the higher forms of reflection.

It might be argued that the learning cycle is for the individual and the audit cycle is for the clinical team. In fact, audit is a group learning task that involves group learning processes and group learning outcomes. It follows that careful

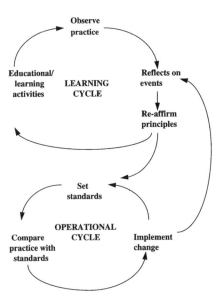

Figure 5.4 The links between the learning and audit cycles

attention to the dynamics and environment of the group are important factors in the success of an audit. Box 5.4 offers some suggestions. Equally important is a recognition of resistances (or obstacles) in the learning and audit cycles and how to reduce them (Box 5.5). Finally, it should be noted that either the learning or the audit cycle may stimulate ideas for research and for the development of new modes of practice.

5.11 LEARNING IN AUDIT

Learning opportunities in the audit cycle occur as shown in the areas A, B, C and D of Figure 5.5.

5.11.1 Stage A

The stimulus may arise from published guidelines, research evidence, the observation of others' practice, untoward events, complaints, purchaser input or proposed clinical service development. The negotiation of standards includes:

- The recognition of the roles of all professionals.
- The views of patients/carers.
- The search for sound research evidence for the development of agreed standards.

Box 5.4   Simple but important suggestions for group audit work

- *Physical* – room size, chairs in a circle/round a table, beverages available, room fittings, overhead projector.
- *Interpersonal* – mutual respect, acceptance of others' strengths and failings, willingness to admit faults without fear of recriminations, opportunity for full discussion.
- *Social* – encouragement of group loyalty, respect for the views of everyone – especially those of junior staff, mutual confidentiality.
- *Culture* – audit activities promoted and valued by the institution, challenge and change promoted, clear aims for health care agreed, openness.
- *Resources* – protected time for audit, audit assistants, journals/books, video, information technology, office/secretarial support etc., readily available.
- *Motivation* – acceptable goals, expectations of success, positive image of audit, desire for enhanced proficiency.

Box 5.5   Reducing resistance to change

Who brings a change?
Resistance is less:
- If those involved feel it is their own project.
- If it has whole-hearted and visible support of the leaders, and the leaders continue to support the project after the initial stages.

What kinds of change?
Resistance is less:
- If the change appeals to values which have long been acknowledged but perhaps neglected.
- If the change is seen as reducing rather than increasing present burdens.
- If the change offers the kinds of new experiences which interest participants.
- If participants feel that their autonomy and security are not threatened.
- If visible efforts are made to maximize gains and minimize losses.

What procedures?
Resistance is less:
- If participants have shares in the evaluation and development and they agree that the problems identified are important.
- If the project is adopted by group consensus.
- If proponents empathize with opponents, recognize and accept valid objections and suggestions and allay unnecessary fears.
- If it is recognized that innovations are often misinterpreted and misunderstood, so patient, clear and perhaps frequent explaining is required. So, too, are opportunities for feedback and further clarification.
- If the project is kept open to revision and re-evaluation.
- If the experience of the participants indicates that changes are desirable.
- If participants support, trust and have confidence in their relations with one another.

(Brown et al, 1997)

The aim here is to ensure that the standards negotiated are both relevant to patient needs and are evidence-based. When negotiating standards, the team need to examine what counts as the objective indicators of good practice. Specific exceptions need to be defined and sources for data concerning these indicators identified. These indicators need to be agreed with all the professional groups involved in the change of practice. All of these tasks require high level critical and reflective learning and, sometimes, consummate social skills.

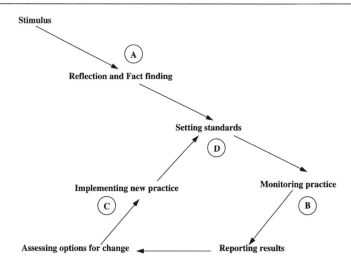

Figure 5.5 Learning opportunities in the audit cycle

5.11.2   Stage B

This stage relates the process of peer review to the consideration of options for change. At the stage of monitoring, the data are collected and analysed and a report prepared for presentation to the peer review meeting. We have already emphasized, in the section on the audit cycle, the importance of the presentation of the report to the peer review meeting. At that meeting, participants should note compliance and non-compliance with standards. It is usually best to begin with a dispassionate consideration of the facts and then explore the attitudes and concerns of the clinical team. Known, surmised and other possible reasons for the cause of problems should also be considered. The diagnosis of any problems found should lead to a consideration of the options for change. The aim is to consider all possible practical options, even those which may have been considered, initially, as impractical. Involvement of general managers in appraising options is advisable, especially if their help will be needed in implementation of change. It may be necessary to consult widely, outside of the clinical team, when considering the options for change. Considering all the options openly, and without bias, is an essential part of the process of learning from audit as well as learning in audit. This stage requires reflective learning, social skills and creative thinking.

5.11.3   Stage C

This stage provides the challenge of translating choices into action. The changes in clinical practice that are planned and implemented may involve educational or operational elements or, more frequently, both. In other words, the audit may have identified learning needs that are necessary for clinical effectiveness which might be fulfilled either in a course or a change in practice. Here again, reflective learning and persuasion are necessary and, in addition, detailed planning.

5.11.4   Stage D

This stage involves moving through the cycle again to ensure that practice has changed towards the agreed standards. At this stage, the learning and development achieved may be the subject of a summative rather than a formative audit.

5.12   A CASE STUDY OF LEARNING IN AUDIT

Patrick Jeffery (personal communication, 1994) allowed Batstone and Edwards (1994) to use his experience of being involved in an audit of breast cancer services. We have told his story with annotations that indicate the kinds of learning being undertaken (Table 5.2). Problem specific learning deals with a specific issue, whereas conceptual learning is more concerned with the assumptions or ideas on which care is based. Deliberate learning refers to the use of independent study and courses, whereas experiential learning is that achieved through reflection on audit findings. Incidental, or opportunistic, learning is learning that was unplanned or unintentional, whereas formal learning has specific known objectives.

This audit led to considerable change in the delivery of service but, more importantly, it modified clinical practice with an emphasis on assessing and meeting patients' needs and feelings. The story also indicates how learning from patients can be used in the clinical audit process.

5.13   LEARNING BASED ON AUDIT

An audit might yield learning needs of an individual, a clinical team, a professional group or even a trust itself. As indicated, group learning is part of the audit process and the group learning itself might well be part of an audit. Box 5.6 offers a possible method of auditing quickly a group's learning processes.

For guidelines to be implemented successfully, one needs to ensure that other groups involved also learn about the new approach. The steps necessary are:

• Dissemination of guidelines to all relevant health care professionals.
• Adaptation to meet local needs.
• Adoption by all health care professionals involved.

Table 5.2   A case study of learning in audit

The audit as it unfolded	Learning aspects of the audit
Patrick, a surgeon who has a special interest in the surgery for treatment of breast cancer, began to consider whether his joint follow-up clinics with a radiotherapist were appreciated by both patients and general practitioners and whether they were worthwhile. An audit of care of patients with breast cancer was conceived and consideration of standards commenced.	Curiosity – conceptual, informal, experiential Literature review – deliberate, problem solving
Whilst attending a national meeting to hear a discussion of risk management, he listened to a lecture about the role of consumers in healthcare given by Marianne Rigge, director of the College of Health. This confirmed his curiosity and extended the area of interest to a much more patient-orientated view of the audit.	Information association – conceptual, informal Elaboration – deliberate, conceptual
Contact was made with the College of Health to learn of their experience in assessing patient perceptions of clinical care. This involved the staff of the audit department and the nurse responsible for promoting the quality of care. At this point, a list of all interested parties was made and Patrick undertook to contact them concerning the audit project. A previous audit of fine needle aspiration had involved histopathologists, who were readily recruited to the new project. Discussions with radiologists and radiographers concentrated thoughts on areas of their work which were relevant and standard setting began. Standards from the national Breast Screening Program were adapted by surgical and nursing staff to suit patients presenting with disease. The radiotherapist concentrated on standards for access to the service whilst pharmacists considered the delivery of chemotherapy.	Communication – deliberate, conceptual, informal Disseminating awareness – deliberate, informal Literature review – deliberate, problem solving Revision of guidelines – deliberate problem solving Consensus standards – deliberate, informal Seeking patient views – deliberate, conceptual
The College of Health undertook semi-structured interviews with patients based on findings from their previous studies. Ethical committee approval had been sought for these interviews, criteria agreed and a patient selection procedure for a retrospective audit undertaken.	Peer review meetings – experiential and deliberate
The findings of the audit were discussed at a number of peer review meetings. The College of Health findings were initially reported to Patrick and the lead audit assistants before being discussed by a wider group including medical, nursing, OPD and quality staff. Other peer groups discussed data relevant to their particular input and proposals discussed within the wider group. From this, an action plan with dates for completion was agreed.	Agreeing change – deliberate, formal, problem solving
Some actions were undertaken immediately in response to patients' views, e.g. suggesting patients brought someone to drive them home because they might find breast aspiration uncomfortable, whilst others required planning, e.g. making pyjamas rather than openback gowns available for mammograms. Some senior staff have attended courses in counselling techniques. Over the next 6 months an agreed programme of improvements was implemented. Further, it was agreed to repeat the audit including the consumer element in 18 months to confirm that learning and change had taken place to find out what new lessons need to be learnt.	Implementing change through explanation – conceptual, deliberate, informal Further learning – formal, deliberate, problem solving Planned review – openness to further possibilities for learning and problem solving

(Based on Batstone and Edwards, 1994)

Box 5.6 A tool to assess the learning processes of an audit group

Most of our meetings were confused	1 2 3 4 5	Most of our meetings were well organized
We often got side-tracked	1 2 3 4 5	We stuck to the task most of the time
We didn't listen to each other	1 2 3 4 5	We did listen to each other
Some talked too much and some did not talk enough	1 2 3 4 5	We all contributed to the discussion
We did not think through our ideas sufficiently	1 2 3 4 5	We thought through our ideas well
Some got aggressive and some got upset	1 2 3 4 5	We were able to argue and discuss without rancour
Most of us seemed to be bored by the discussion	1 2 3 4 5	Most of us seemed to enjoy the discussion
Most of us did not improve our discussion skills	1 2 3 4 5	Most of us did improve our discussion skills
Most of us did not learn much	1 2 3 4 5	Most of us did learn through our group work

Note: the discussion is more important than the rating.
How could your group have worked better?
(Brown et al, 1997)

- Implementation of modified practice.
- Monitoring the process of change.
- Evaluating the outcomes.

All of these tasks involve learning. The first two stages are predominantly learning tasks, whilst the third and fourth are also part of change management and the last two are predominantly clinical audits of process and outcomes.

Finally, after an audit, participants should meet to reflect upon what they have learnt from the processes and outcomes of audit. The reflections might encompass social as well as cognitive learning.

5.14   LEARNING FOR AUDIT

Audit requires skills derived from social science as well as clinical skills. Until clinical audit is part of the curriculum of the basic training of all health care professionals, there is a major task in training existing staff to undertake audit projects. In particular, methods of monitoring practice, the negotiation and articulation of standards and the skills of persuasive presentation require careful attention. For medical staff, there has been the stimulus of Royal Colleges requiring evidence of clinical audit in their review of posts for doctors in training. Accreditation of clinical pathology services has similarly required evidence of participation in clinical audit. The organizational audit of the King's Fund takes a similar approach. Audit is also recognized by the regulatory body of nurses, midwives and health visitors, as part of continuing professional development for re-registration.

Initial audit training is usually undertaken in single profession speciality groups. Our experience, like that of many others, is that courses in audit techniques are best organized as two sessions separated by a period of 4–6 weeks during which the participants undertake a simple audit of their own team or department. This bases the training firmly in the participants' workplaces and, it gives them an opportunity to develop and share their growing expertise in audit.

When audit training is organized for multi-professional groups, it is our experience that a substantial session on team working and team building needs to be incorporated in the programme in order that individuals recognize and value the various roles that different professionals play. Different courses are required for those who intend to lead clinical audit for speciality groups or clinical directorates. These need to emphasize ways of helping individuals and groups to deal with change and learn from their audit findings. For audit support staff, a wide variety of training courses may be needed, including the use of information technology, negotiation, assertiveness, persuasion, presentation skills, statistical analysis and clinical audit techniques (Robertson et al, 1996).

Such training for audit is necessary, but it is not the whole story. Whenever an audit is to be undertaken by a clinical team, they need to prepare and plan carefully for it. Indeed, much learning and critical thinking can, and should, take place in the early stages of planning for an audit.

5.15 SUMMARY POINTS

Within the complex relations of clinical audit and learning some key points emerge:

- Audit is a genus of assessment. It is essentially a learning rather than a managerial tool but it requires an impetus for learning, a desire for improvement, a quest for excellence.
- The nature and purposes of the audit process and cycle need to be understood so that people can use audit effectively.

- Audit is a method of learning as well as a method of assessment.
- All the perspectives of learning have something to offer to the processes of audit and the audit cycle. The key component is learning based upon experiences and reflection.
- There are intimate links between the cycle of audit and the cycle of reflective learning.
- Reflective learning in audit, on audit and for audit are important features of the audit process.
- Sensitivity to the values and beliefs of the group is important particularly during the planning stages of audit and the presentation of audit results.
- In addition, clinicians will need to develop and use team leadership skills to create those improvements in quality care that are indicated by audit findings. Often, they may need to seek the help and cooperation of general managers.
- Audit provides opportunities for individuals, clinical teams, specialist subgroups, trusts and education committees to exploit the opportunities arising from audit.
- Finally, audit poses an exciting challenge for those interested in developing the quality of clinical care at all levels. It provides different approaches to learning in the work place and it offers a firm ground for the development of courses based upon needs-analyses obtained in the process of clinical audit.

REFERENCES

Ausubel D (1989) *Educational Psychology: A Cognitive View*. Second edition. New York: Holt, Rinehart & Winston.

Batstone GF and Edwards M (1994) Managing of learning and professional development through audit. In: White T (editor) *Textbook of Management for Doctors*. London: Churchill Livingstone.

Beckard R and Pritchard W (1992) *Changing the Essence: the Art of Creating and Leading Fundamental Change in Organisations*. San Francisco: Jossey Bass.

Boud D et al (1995) *Enhancing Learning through Self Assessment*. London: Kogan Page.

Boud D, Keogh R and Walker M (1985) *Reflection: Turning Experience in to Learning*. London: Kogan Page.

Brewin CR (1988) *Cognitive Foundations of Clinical Psychology*. London: Lawrence Erlbaum Associates.

Brookfield SD (1986) *Understanding and Facilitating Adult Learning*. Buckingham: Open University Press.

Brown G, Bull J and Pendlebury M (1997) *Assessing Student Learning in Higher Education*. London: Routledge.

Clarke K (1990) Speech to the joint meeting of the National Association of Clinical Tutors, the Conference of Postgraduate Deans and the National Association of Postgraduate Centre Administrators. York, 6 July 1990.

Cowan J (1998) *Supporting the Reflective Learner*. Buckingham: Open University Press.

Department of Health (1994) *The Evolution of Clinical Audit*. Leeds: NHS Executive.

Entwistle NJ (1987) *Styles of Learning and Teaching*. Second edition. Chichester: Wiley.

Entwistle NJ (1992) *The Impact of Teaching on Learning Outcomes*. Sheffield: USDU/CVCP.

Falchikov N (1996) *Improving Learning Through Critical Peer Feedback and Reflection*. HERDSA Conference papers, Perth, Western Australia.

Falchikov N and Boud D (1989) Student Self Assessment in higher education: a meta analysis. *Review of Educational Research* 59:395–430.

Frostick SP and Wallace A (eds) *Medical Audit*. Cambridge: Cambridge University Press.

Handy C (1993) *Understanding Organisations*. Harmondsworth: Penguin Books.

Hatton N and Smith D (1995) Reflection: towards definition and implementation. *Teaching and Teacher Education* 11:33–51.

Heath R (1964) *The Reasonable Adventurer*. Pittsburgh: University of Pittsburgh Press.

Hilgard ER (1962) *Theories of Learning*. New York: Methuen

Honey P and Mumford A (1983) *Using your Learning Styles*. Maidenhead: Peter Honey.

Knowles MS (1990) *The Adult Learner: A Neglected Species*. Second edition. Houston: Gulf Publishing Company.

Kolb D (1976) *Learning Style Inventory: Technical Manual*. Boston: McBer.

Kolb D (1984) *Experiential Learning: Experience as a Source of Learning*. Englewood Cliffs: Prentice Hall.

Lough JRM and Murray TS (1997) Teaching audit – lessons from summative assessment. *Br J Gen Pract* 47:829–830.

Marinker M (1990) *Medical Audit and General Practice*. London: MSD/British Medical Journal.

Maslow AH (1973) *The Farther Reaches of Human Nature*. Harmondsworth: Penguin Books.

Mitchell L and Cuthbert T (1989) *Insufficient Evidence; The Final Report of the Competency Testing Project*. Glasgow: SCOTVEC Project.

Norman D (1980) Cognitive Engineering in Education. In: Tumo DJ and Reis S (editors). *Problem Solving and Education*. Hillsdale, New Jersey: Lawrence Erlbaum.

Perry WG (1981) *Forms of Intellectual and Ethical Development in the College Years*. New York: Holt Rinehart Winston.

Pettigrew A, Ferlie E and McKee L (1992) *Shaping Strategic Change in Large Organisations: The Case of the NHS*. London: Sage.

Piaget J and Inhelder B (1969) *The Psychology of The Child*. London: Routledge.

Power M (1994) *The Audit Explosion*. London: Demos, Paper 7.

Robertson N, Hearnshaw HM and Baker R (1996) Development and evaluation of a course for audit support staff in primary care. *J Clin Effect* 1:137–140.

Rogers CR (1969) *Freedom to Learn*. Columbus, Ohio: Charles E. Merrill.

Rogers CR (1983) *Freedom to Learn in the 80's*. Columbus, Ohio: Charles E. Merrill.

Roth I (1990) (editor) *Introduction to Psychology* (Volumes 1 and 2). Hove: Lawrence Erlbaum Associates (with the Open University).

Royal College of Physicians (1989) *Medical Audit; a First Report. What, How and Why?* London: Royal College of Physicians.

Royal College of Surgeons (1989) *Guidelines to Clinical Audit in Surgical Practice*. London: Royal College of Surgeons.

Schmidt HG, Norman GR and Boshuzen HPA (1990) A cognitive perspective on medical expertise: theory and implications. *Academic Medicine* 65:611–621.

Schon DA (1983) *The Reflective Practitioner*. London: Temple Smith.

Schon DA (1988) *Educating the Reflective Practitioner*. San Francisco: Jossey-Bass.

SCOPME (1989) *Medical Audit: The Educational Implications*. London: Standing Committee of Postgraduate and Continuing Education.

Stevens R (1990) Humanistic psychology. In: Roth I (editor) *Introduction to Psychology*. Hove: Lawrence Erlbaum Associates (with the Open University).

Vygotsky LR (1962) *Thought and Language*. Massachusetts: MIT Press.

Wittrock M (1986) *Students Thought Processes*. In: Wittrock M (editor) *Handbook of Research on Teaching*. New York: Macmillan.

Chapter 6

AUDIT ACROSS INTERFACES[1]

M. P. Eccles, M. Deverill, E. McColl, J. Newton and J. Verrill

6.1 INTRODUCTION

Health care in the UK NHS is clearly divided into primary and secondary care, and there is only limited face-to-face contact between health care professionals from the two sectors. In contrast, patients frequently move both backwards and forwards across the interface between the two sectors. Certain elements of the structure, process and outcome of care that patients receive attain greater prominence as they move backwards and forwards. At its best, movement between the sectors will be 'seamless', with the care of a patient totally coordinated as they move from their own home, via primary care services into secondary care and back again. At its worst, care at the interface may suffer from problems such as inadequate sharing of relevant information about patients, and unplanned discharge from, or readmission to, secondary care. The process of care for clinical conditions for which patients require referral, the referral process itself, and communication across the primary–secondary care interface, all have the potential to affect the quality of the care that patients receive. For that reason, they form legitimate topics for audit.

Although there is no clear consensus, 'interface audit' has been defined by Baker (1994), as *'complete audit cycles* conducted by *professionals from both primary and secondary care* working together as a team to *improve quality'* (our italics). There are three important facets to this definition. Firstly, interface audit, in common with other types of audit, is deemed to have successfully occurred only if all stages within the audit cycle, including change and re-evaluation, have been completed. Secondly, there must be active involvement of both sides of the primary–secondary interface. One-way audits of activity across

---

[1]This chapter is based on articles originally published in *Audit Trends* 1995; **3(4)**:127–131 and *Quality in Health Care*, 1996; **5**:193–200 and has been published with the permission of the journal editors.

---

the interface are specifically excluded; these can be more judgemental than useful (Bryce et al, 1990) and are limited in their effectiveness, since changes identified by one side or the other are unlikely to be implemented. Finally, audit should seek to improve quality of care.

While the main aim is quality improvement, there may be additional benefits. Collaborating in an audit will bring together groups of health care professionals who might not otherwise meet, thus providing the potential for interchange on a broader range of topics, and for improved communication and understanding between the two sectors of the health service. However, Baker (1994), in his analysis of interface audit, is not optimistic about current practice suggesting that, whilst one-way audit and quality assessment projects are commonplace, *bona fide* interface audits are rare. Moreover, there appears to be little systematically gathered data on audit activity across the primary–secondary care interface.

Much audit activity, whether within a single sector or across disciplines, involves the convening and running of small groups. A large body of literature exists within the fields of sociology and psychology on behaviour in small groups (Brown, 1988; Levine and Moreland, 1990; Diedrich and Dye, 1992; see Chapter 7). A number of issues have been drawn from this literature to inform the effective use of small groups in clinical audit (Scott and Marinker, 1990; Irvine and Irvine, 1991). These have included structural factors such as group size and group task, and process factors such as leadership, communication and role allocation. While these issues can be problematic enough within a single discipline (Newton et al, 1992), group work involving more than one discipline can, because of differing backgrounds and perceptions, potentially exacerbate these problems.

In order to highlight the factors that may influence the implementation of change with interface audit, in this chapter we describe two studies that used different methods to explore issues within audit activity across the interface between primary and secondary care in England and Wales. In the first study, which forms the first section of this chapter, the objectives were: to document the focus of current audit activity across the primary–secondary care interface; to explore participants' experiences of undertaking such audit; to identify factors associated with these experiences; and to gather views on possible future audit activities, and the means by which such audits could be fostered. The second study was a case study examining one group's experience of interface audit work. The group studied had experienced difficulties completing the audit cycle, and by conducting individual interviews with group members on their views of the group's functioning and their perceptions of problems encountered, we hoped to draw out general lessons for the group itself as well as other groups conducting interface audits.

6.2   A NATIONAL SURVEY OF AUDIT ACTIVITY ACROSS THE PRIMARY–SECONDARY CARE INTERFACE

A three-phase national postal questionnaire survey was initiated in mid-1993 using a cascade sampling approach. This technique is similar to the snowball technique used in interview surveys, and uses respondents to each round of the

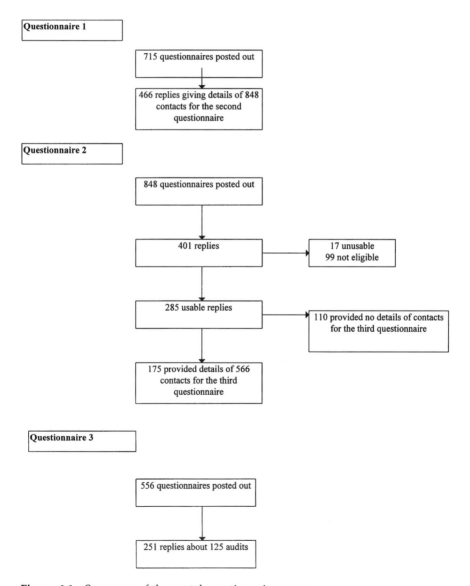

Figure 6.1   Summary of the postal questionnaire survey

Box 6.1   The methods used in the national survey of interface audit

The first questionnaire was posted in June 1993. It asked for brief details of complete or ongoing interface audits and the names and addresses of appropriate contacts. It was sent to groups and individuals identified through previous networking, as well as medical audit advisory group (MAAG) and medical audit committee (MAC) chairs, medical audit facilitators, directors of public health, academic departments of general practice, regional advisers in general practice, Royal College of General Practitioners faculty secretaries and health authority general managers. The responses were used to generate the list of recipients for second phase questionnaires.

The second questionnaire was sent out in October 1993. It gathered details about the audit topic and the structure and organization of the audit group (Box 6.2). Respondents were asked to supply the names and addresses of all their interface audit group members.

All those thus identified were sent the third questionnaire in January 1994. This gathered information about individual group members, their opinions of participating in an interface audit and their views on subsequent interface audit activity (Box 6.3).

In two questions within the third questionnaire (questions four and five), respondents were asked to answer on a five-point Likert scale (strongly agree to strongly disagree). Six open ended questions (questions 8, 9, 11, 12, 13 and 14) examined the lessons learnt from participating in an interface audit, the impact of working with people known previously, suggested topics for future audits and the factors which would facilitate and encourage interface audit in the future. These responses were read, common themes were identified and codes were developed and applied.

The data were analysed using the Statistical Package for Social Sciences (SPSS, 1990). The χ^2 test was used to test the significance of associations. Where a linear trend in percentage agreement was expected (e.g. with respect to group size and length of meeting), the Mantel–Haenzel χ^2 was used (Mantel and Haenzel, 1959).

survey to generate the sampling frame for the subsequent round. In each phase, a single reminder (including a duplicate questionnaire) was sent to non-responders after 3 weeks. The phases of the survey are summarized in Figure 6.1. The methods are summarized in Box 6.1, and full details can be found in Eccles et al (1996a).

To examine whether subjective experiences of interface audit were related to characteristics of the audit itself and of the group, factual data from the second

---

Box 6.2   Summary of questionnaire 2: details of audits taking place at the interface between primary and secondary care

1. What was the title of the audit?
2. Which categories were covered by the audit? (explicit list)
3. What was the trigger for initiating the audit? (explicit list)
4. Which steps of the audit cycle has the group covered? (explicit list)
5. What type of group was involved with the audit? (explicit list)
6. Which specialities were represented in the audit group? (explicit list)
7. Which specialities provided input for the audit without being part of the group? (explicit list)
8. How many people were there in the audit group altogether?
9. Who initiated the audit?
10. What was the status of the initiator?
11. What was the initiator's role in the audit group?
12. Did the audit involve setting explicit guidelines for care or performance?
13. Who was involved in setting guidelines? (explicit list)
14. Was a literature search carried out?
15. Who undertook the data collection? (explicit list)
16. Have the data been analysed?
17. Who analysed the data? (explicit list)
18. Is the audit now complete?
19. How long did it take? OR
20. How long has the audit been taking place for up to now?
21. At what time of day did the meetings usually take place?
22. How long did meetings usually last?
23. How frequently did the groups meet?
24. How many meetings have been held to date?
25. Where were the meetings held?
26. Did the audit require funding?
27. Where did the funding come from?

---

questionnaire and experiential information from the third questionnaire were combined. We considered three specific areas:

- Who initiated the audit: we hypothesized that collaboratively initiated audits, with input from both primary and secondary care, would be more successful (Bryce et al, 1990; Baker, 1994).
- Length of meetings: lack of time for audit is often offered as a reason for not participating in audit activity (Spencer, 1993; McColl et al, 1994) so we tested whether length of meeting was associated with views of success.

Box 6.3   Summary of questionnaire 3: experiences of audits taking place at the interface between primary and secondary care

1. What was the topic of the audit which involved both primary and secondary care?
2. Please indicate your status (explicit list).
3. Did you have a specific role within the group and if so what?
4. Listed below are some statements relating to group work: to what extent do you feel the following statements are true of your experiences within the interface audit group?
   a. The task of the group was well understood.
   b. The task of the group was accepted by its members.
   c. There was a high level of participation in the group.
   d. The group took no longer than necessary to complete its tasks.
   e. Every idea was given a hearing.
   f. There were few disagreements in the group.
   g. Any disagreements were effectively resolved.
   h. Decisions reflected a consensus of group opinion.
   i. The group enjoyed the experience of working together.
5. Listed below are some statements about interface audit: to what extent do you feel the following statements are true of your experiences within the interface audit group?
   a. The group provided a forum for discussion relating to aspects of care other than the audit topic.
   b. A number of possible topics for another interface audit were discussed.
   c. The meetings led to closer working relations between primary and secondary care.
   d. The meetings provided clinicians from both primary and secondary care with the opportunity to discuss areas of common concern.
   e. Meetings stimulated learning.
   f. Group members enjoyed meeting colleagues, especially those from another discipline.
   g. Finding somewhere neutral for the meetings was a problem.
   h. There was disagreement over who should be responsible for funding the audit.
   i. Deciding who should be responsible for data collection was a problem.
   j. Identifying which party should be responsible for the analysis was a problem.
   k. There was disagreement about the ownership of the data.
   l. Confidentiality of data between primary and secondary care was an issue.

continues

— continued —

    m. It was difficult to establish common goals between the different
       parties to the audit.
    n. The computer systems between primary and secondary care were
       not compatible.
    o. The physical distance between group members created problems.
 6. If you had known what the experience of interface audit would be like
    before this audit would you still have participated?
 7. Would you participate in another interface audit in the future?
 8. What were the main lessons learnt from the experience?
 9. Would you do anything differently if you had another chance and if so
    what?
10. Did you know any of the other members of the group before the audit?
11. Did you think this was helpful to the group work?
12. Why/why not? (to clarify 11)
13. What interface audit topics would be of interest to you in the future?
14. What do you consider would be important factors in facilitating interface
    audit in the future?
15. What do you think would encourage more audit to take place at the
    interface between primary and secondary care?

- Group size and composition: size has often been seen as crucial to the way
  in which an audit group operates and has been a reason for highlighting the
  importance of having a skilled small group leader (Eccles et al, 1996b). Scott
  and Marinker (1990) see groups that are too small as limiting creativity and
  allowing strong personalities to dominate, whilst too large a group leads to
  erosion of cohesion; they suggest that eight is the optimum number. Larger
  groups have been seen as not operating as well as smaller groups (of about
  seven people) (Firth Cozens, 1992); large groups may also lead to practical
  difficulties, for example in arranging meetings. While it will be possible to
  conduct interface audits within a small group, interface groups are more
  likely than non-interface groups to be large and we wanted to explore the
  consequences both of this and of the effect of previously knowing other
  group members.

6.3 RESULTS

Information about the respondents and response rates is included in Box 6.4.
Topic areas covered by the audits are shown in Table 6.1. When allowance was
made for audits covering more than one area, 56% contained some element of

---

Box 6.4   The respondents in the national survey of interface audit

The first questionnaire was sent to 715 contacts and generated 466 replies (response rate 65%). These produced 848 contacts for the second question-naire, from whom 401 questionnaires were returned (response rate 47%). However, 17 were unusable and a further 99 did not fit the definition of interface audit (Baker, 1994), leaving a usable sample size of 285. Of the 285 valid responses to the second questionnaire, 175 provided contact details for their group members; this gave 556 names for the third questionnaire. From these, we obtained 251 replies (response rate 45%) reporting on 125 audits. The median response rate per reported audit was 47% (the number of respondents ranged from zero to five). In both the second and third question-naires, item non-response rates varied from question to question. Therefore, where the number of respondents to a given question was less than that for the corresponding questionnaire as a whole, the appropriate denominator is given in the text and tables.

Forty-seven percent of respondents (119) to the third questionnaire were pri-mary care based, 46% (116) were from secondary care, 4% (10) were from public health and 2% (6) came from other sectors or were in posts spanning sectors. The largest number of respondents were doctors [139 of 251 (55%)]; 78 (31%) of those were general practitioner principals and 61 (24%) were hospital doctors.

---

patient/disease management. Thirty-three percent of the audits were within a single area; 27% within two; 19% within three; and 21% covered four or more topic areas.

6.3.1   Initiation of the audit

In a question asking about the trigger for initiating the audit, it was possible to give more than one response; therefore, the percentages total more than 100%. Most audits had more than one trigger. For 61% (170/277) of respondents, a perceived problem was at least part of the reason for undertaking audit; for 58% the topic was of mutual interest but only 9% of respondents endorsed economic reasons as a trigger. Only 18% of audits were initiated collaboratively, with primary care initiating 39% and secondary care initiating 33%. Management or other groups were responsible for initiation in 10% of cases. The majority of initiators were doctors (178/247; 72% of audits); the only other sizeable cate-gory of staff initiating audits was audit support personnel (41; 17%).

Table 6.1 Areas covered by interface audits (n = 276) (Questionnaire 2; question 2)

Topics	% (number of audits)
Patient/disease management only	15 (40)
Referral only	4 (10)
Discharge only	4 (11)
Communications only	5 (14)
Use of secondary resources only	3 (9)
One other only	3 (7)
Patient/disease management + any one of other above categories	42 (115)
Other combinations of two or more categories	25 (69)

6.3.2 Composition of audit groups

The majority of audits (178/283; 63%) involved collaborative groups set up specifically to conduct the audit, with primary health care medical audit advisory groups (MAAGs) involved in 52% of audits and hospital medical audit committees (MACs) in 33%. The majority of groups (58%) had between three and eight members. While groups of two were rare (5%), groups of nine to 11 (14%) and 12 or more (23%) were not uncommon. The representation of health care professions within interface audit groups is shown in Table 6.2.

As with initiation, doctors dominated. The next largest groups were primary and secondary care audit support staff. The total number of disciplines per audit ranged from two to 19. Approximately 30% (85) of audits had an equal number of primary and secondary specialities.

6.3.3 Involvement in tasks within the audit

In terms of task allocation, we asked about who was involved in setting guidelines, data collection and data analysis. We also asked who had input into the audit without being a group member. While the setting of guidelines was highly doctor dominated, the largest share of data collection (by percentage of audits) was undertaken by audit support staff in secondary care – 42% (105/252) of audits (Table 6.2). Data analysis was dominated by secondary (44%) and primary (31%) care audit support staff.

6.3.4 Length of meetings

For 48% of the groups, the average duration of meetings was less than 1 h; for 28%, meetings generally lasted 60–90 min, while for the remaining 24% the average meeting took over 90 min.

Table 6.2 Representation of health care professions within interface audit groups: overall; in setting guidelines; and in data collection. (Percentages do not add up to 100 because of representation of multiple professions in groups and activities)

Health care profession	% (number) of audits in which each was represented		
	Overall representation ($n = 285$)	Setting guidelines ($n = 158$)	Data collection ($n = 252$)
Secondary care			
Hospital doctor	90 (257)	83 (131)	24 (61)
Hospital nurse/midwife	28 (79)	21 (33)	10 (24)
Hospital manager	15 (43)	9 (14)	2 (6)
Hospital professions allied to medicine	27 (77)	30 (47)	7 (17)
Audit support staff	59 (167)	22 (35)	42 (105)
Others	22 (63)	19 (30)	17 (42)
Primary care			
GP principal	92 (262)	82 (129)	38 (96)
Practice nurse	18 (52)	13 (21)	11 (27)
Community nurse/midwife	20 (58)	10 (15)	6 (16)
Practice manager/receptionist	17 (48)	4 (7)	23 (58)
Community professions allied to medicine	14 (40)	16 (25)	3 (7)
Audit support staff	41 (116)	18 (29)	27 (69)
Others	25 (72)	17 (26)	12 (31)

6.3.5   Progress round the audit cycle

The questionnaire set out nine steps of the audit cycle (Lawrence, 1993) and Table 6.3 shows how many of these steps were completed by audits that were reportedly complete, reportedly in progress or incomplete. Of completed audits, almost all had collected and analysed data relating to practice after standards had been set or agreed. Three-quarters had suggested changes, but only two-fifths had implemented change and only a quarter had evaluated change.

6.3.6   Experiences of interface audit

There were widespread feelings of successful group working, as indicated in Table 6.4.

With respect to experiences of interface audit (Table 6.5), whilst none of the statements show unanimity, most reflect a positive view (for those statements

Table 6.3 Percentage (number) of audits completing steps of the audit cycle by whether the audit was reported to be complete or not

Step	Audit 'complete' (n = 117)	Audit 'incomplete' (n = 154)	All audits (n = 271)
1. Observe practice	90% (105)	84% (130)	87% (235)
2. Set/adapt standards	78% (91)	75% (115)	76% (206)
3. Collect data	99% (116)	92% (141)	95% (257)
4. Analysis of data	98% (115)	68% (105)	81% (220)
5. Compare practice to standard	76% (89)	40% (62)	56% (151)
6. Suggest change	74% (87)	47% (73)	59% (160)
7. Implement change	39% (46)	27% (42)	33% (88)
8. Evaluate change	25% (29)	12% (19)	18% (48)
9. Review standard/re-audit	22% (26)	10% (15)	15% (41)

phrased in a negative manner low percentage responses indicate positive views).

Only one-quarter to one-third of respondents did not agree with the three statements: 'Meetings provided clinicians from both primary and secondary care with the opportunity to discuss areas of common concern'; 'Group members enjoyed meeting colleagues, especially those from another discipline'; and 'Meetings stimulated learning'. However, 38% did not agree with the statement 'Meetings led to closer working relations between primary and secondary care'. Infrastructure barriers were also identified, in particular problems with incompatible computer systems.

6.3.7   Factors influencing views of interface audit

6.3.7.1   Length of meetings

At least 90% of respondents felt that the 'task of the group was well understood'. The longer the meeting, the higher the percentage agreeing with this statement: 96% (65/68) in groups whose meetings lasted over 90 min; 93% (86/93) for groups with meetings of 60–90 min duration; and 84% (73/87) for groups whose meetings lasted less than 60 min (χ^2 for trend = 6.23, $p = 0.01$). Length of meeting was also significantly associated with positive responses regarding high levels of participation. Similarly, the longer the meeting the greater the opportunity for discussion of topics of common concern. However, it seems possible that some groups' meetings may have been protracted by discussion of issues of data confidentiality. Only 7% (6/83) of respondents from groups with short meetings agreed that 'Confidentiality of data between primary and secondary care was an issue', compared to 15%

Table 6.4 Percentage (*n/N*) of respondents positively endorsing statements about experiences of interface audit group work

Statement	% agree + strongly agree (*n/N*)
The task of the group was well understood	90% (225/250)
The task of the group was accepted by its members	90% (225/250)
Decisions reflected a consensus of group opinion	84% (208/247)
Every idea was given a hearing	81% (201/248)
The group enjoyed the experience of working together	80% (199/248)
Any disagreements were effectively resolved	78% (184/237)
There was a high level of participation	76% (190/249)
There were few disagreements in the group	71% (177/248)
The group took no longer than necessary to complete its tasks	63% (154/246)

(13/87) from medium length meetings and 19% (13/67) from the longest meetings ($p = 0.03$).

6.3.7.2   Initiation of audit

Joint initiation of an audit appeared to facilitate greater understanding of the group task; 98% (48/49) of respondents from audits initiated collaboratively were in agreement with the statement 'the task of the group was well understood'. The corresponding figures for secondary- and primary-initiated audits were 92% (66/72) and 88% (98/111), respectively ($\chi^2 = 11.97, p = 0.007$). Audits initiated solely by someone without the primary or secondary care sectors were more likely to experience problems with data confidentiality (6/16; 38%); the corresponding figures for primary-initiated, secondary-initiated and collaboratively-initiated audits were 11% (12/108), 12% (8/68) and 13% (6/45), respectively ($p = 0.04$).

6.3.7.3   Group size and composition

Not surprisingly, the larger the group conducting the interface audit, the greater the opportunity for primary and secondary care specialists to discuss matters of common concern. Group size also influenced the likelihood of disagreement within the group, although there was no significant linear trend. Eighty-three percent of people (57/69) in groups of two to five felt that there had been few disagreements as against 65% (51/78) in groups of six to eight and 68% (69/101) in groups of nine or more (χ^2 for trend, $p = 0.05$).

In the third questionnaire, respondents were also asked to indicate whether they had known other members of the group prior to the audit. Ninety percent of respondents (226/250) had prior knowledge of at least one other group

Table 6.5 Percentage (*n*/N) of respondents positively endorsing statements about experiences of working across the interface

Statement	% agree + strongly agree (*n*/N)
Meetings provided clinicians from both primary and secondary care with the opportunity to discuss areas of common concern	79% (193/245)
Group members enjoyed meeting colleagues, especially those from another discipline	77% (184/238)
Meetings stimulated learning	69% (173/250)
The group provided a forum for discussion relating to aspects of care other than the audit topic	66% (162/244)
The computer systems between primary and secondary care were not compatible	62% (79/127)
Meetings led to closer working relations between primary and secondary care	62% (154/248)
A number of possible topics for another interface audit were discussed	57% (132/231)
The physical distance between group members created problems	23% (56/240)
It was difficult to establish common goals between the different parties to the audit	19% (46/247)
Confidentiality of data between primary and secondary care was an issue	13% (32/239)
There was disagreement over who should be responsible for funding the audit	11% (23/201)
Finding somewhere neutral for the meetings was a problem	10% (23/231)
Deciding who should be responsible for data collection was a problem	9% (21/242)
There was disagreement about the ownership of the data	8% (20/244)
Identifying which party should be responsible for the analysis was a problem	8% (20/238)

member. Of these, 95% thought that this was helpful to the way the group worked. A total of 197 respondents gave reasons for their answers, with some mentioning more than one reason. Prior knowledge of other group members was said to lead to good working relationships (29%), efficiency (25%), shared understanding (25%) and trust (24%).

6.3.8 Lessons learnt for the future of interface audit

In an open-ended question, respondents were asked to state the main lessons learnt from their experience; 203 (81%) questionnaires contained responses to this question. The main themes identified were: the importance of setting clear objectives (27%); the importance of primary–secondary communication (20%); the importance of primary–secondary understanding (16%); the need for adequate resources (13%); and the importance of multi-disciplinary working (12%). When asked, in a further open-ended question, what they would do differently in a future interface audit, 34% (54/159) said they would not do anything differently. However, 50 of the 105 who would make some changes said they would ensure that objectives were more clearly specified, 25 would make organizational changes and 24 would aim to improve communications. In response to the question 'If you had known what the experience of interface audit would be like before this audit, would you still have participated?' 94% (235/251) said that they would. Ninety-six percent of all respondents (242/251) stated that they would participate in another interface audit in the future.

6.3.9   Future interface audit activities

Five topics dominated as favourites for future interface audit: referrals/admissions (45/179; 25%); management of chronic diseases (44; 25%); discharge procedures (30; 17%); communications and the management of specific conditions (both 20; 11%). These represent the areas where primary and secondary care are most likely to meet and reflect current interface audit activities (cf. Table 6.1). In answer to open-ended questions about factors that would facilitate future interface activity, and factors that would encourage interface audit activity to take place in the future, the most common responses were commitment, money, time and improved communication (Table 6.6).

Table 6.6   Main factors facilitating future interface audit and encouraging more interface audit. (Questionnaire 3; questions 14 and 15). (Respondents could endorse more than one factor, therefore the total is greater than 100%)

	% of respondents
Factors facilitating future interface audit	
Commitment/enthusiasm	25% (52/208)
Money	24% (50/208)
Time	21% (44/208)
Clear purpose	21% (43/208)
Manpower	17% (36/208)
Improved communications	15% (31/208)
Common objectives	13% (26/208)
Factors encouraging more interface audit	
Money	27% (57/210)
Improved communications	21% (44/210)
Evidence of benefit	20% (43/210)
Time	20% (41/210)
Manpower	10% (20/210)

6.4   A CASE STUDY OF AN INTERFACE AUDIT GROUP

The questionnaire investigation indicated that many issues might influence the impact of interface audit. We explored some of these issues through a case study of one group. This audit group had been convened to address procedures for the discharge of elderly patients from a district general hospital. The minutes of the group's early meetings identified three areas of interest: the workloads of different professionals involved with patients aged 75 years and over, both before and after discharge from hospital; communication between professionals involved with elderly patients, both before and after discharge from hospital; and patient and carer opinions of discharge procedures. Initially formed from a pre-existing multi-disciplinary Elderly Task Force group, a number of other practitioners were recruited to the audit group that was eventually composed of a health and social needs assessment facilitator, a social worker, consultant geriatricians, a secondary care nurse manager, general practitioners, research support staff and a medical audit advisory group coordinator. The initial round of the audit cycle was scheduled to be completed within 6 months but 1 year on, the group were 6 months behind schedule, with no signs of completing the audit cycle.

Twelve of the 13 group members at the time of this study agreed to be interviewed; one group member (a general practitioner) declined. These methods are described in Box 6.5.

6.4.1   The experiences of the group

The group was large, exceeding 12 members on the occasions when there was full attendance; many members cited the size of the group as a problem.

> *I think a smaller group is always easier to work with. I must admit I had difficulty remembering faces [Nurse Manager]*

> *The group was just too big, it really was. There were two or three people who would always have something to say and the majority of the rest of them had nothing to say at all [GP]*

The group encountered further difficulties owing to the fluctuating nature of group membership, which changed throughout the project. This impeded the group process by disrupting continuity and hindering the development of a sense of group identity.

> *There were all sorts of people who sort of popped into the group. There were often people who came and went and nobody was quite sure who all of them were. [GP]*

> *It just looked like any agency in the world that had anything to do with health care was sending a representative [Consultant Geriatrician]*

Box 6.5   Methods used in the case study of the interface audit group

Given that little has been written about the field of interface audit, it was clearly not possible to anticipate all the issues that might arise. Therefore, the interviews were not based around a structured schedule but were guided by a number of key issues highlighted in the existing literature on group work. This left respondents as free as possible to highlight the issues most important to them.

Interviews lasted up to 45 min and were tape recorded and subsequently transcribed. Codes were applied to the transcriptions to highlight common issues which had been raised within the interviews, e.g. comments relating to group size, group task etc. Comments on each issue were collated in order to provide a summary of the group's views on that issue (Miles and Huberman, 1984). The results are presented within a framework for analysing groups (Krech et al, 1962) which assumes that the 'givens' of a group influence the processes within a group which in turn combine to affect the outcome of group activity. The 'givens' of the group were the group members, the nature of the group task and the context within which the group activity was performed. As this latter given runs throughout the whole process, it was not addressed separately. The processes were the interaction between group members, the approach the group took towards the task and the leadership style adopted. The outcomes of group activity were completion of the group task, or productivity, satisfaction and learning on behalf of group members.

The group did not appear to have a clearly defined group task to which all members were committed. It also appears that the project expanded beyond the limits of the resources available to complete the project.

> *I must admit at the start I was a bit unsure exactly what the aim of the group was. I think it became apparent that they were quite confused about exactly what they were looking at [GP]*

> *I think we bit off more than we could chew [Health and Social Needs Facilitator]*

The audit group brought together practitioners who operate at different levels of a traditionally hierarchical environment, e.g. nurses and consultants. This appeared to have inhibited the participation of some group members, who viewed themselves as junior in status to other group members.

> *The medical model isn't about negotiation. It's a power hierarchy. If you're a consultant not many people say 'no' to you. [Health and Social Needs Facilitator]*

> *One of the consultants seemed to have a lot to say. The community nurses seemed to have very little to say at all [Research Assistant]*

Differing professional backgrounds also caused problems; there appeared to be particular problems with involving social services in addition to health care professionals. Issues raised in the interviews included 'language barriers'; lack of knowledge about the practices and systems of other agencies; and complications caused by differing geographical boundaries.

> Social services speak a completely different language to us and we kept having to go back and say, I don't understand what you mean by such a phrase. [GP]

The interviews also indicated that interaction within the group was impeded by concerns that the interests of all members were not being served equally; a sense of mistrust and suspicion was alluded to.

> Well it's been interesting: it hasn't been particularly easy. I think sometimes some of them actually felt a bit threatened by it, but nobody was on a witch hunt, everybody was just really trying to find out the easiest way of cooperating with each other. [GP]

> I know some of the problems (of multi-disciplinary work), some of them are political, very political. Audit should be something that everybody should be involved in. I tended to think that people who were being audited didn't know what was happening. [Nurse Manager]

The approach to the task was highlighted as an issue when a split developed within the group between those members who felt that patients should be consulted and those who felt such consultation was not a valid measure of patient experience. The divide appeared to be along professional boundaries and led to the formation of sub-groups to deal with task completion.

> When I first came I felt the patient perspective was valued by half of the group and the other half were a bit unsure as to what value they could get from that [Research Assistant]

> The comments from the hospital doctors tended to be that patients don't listen. To some extent I think they were 'poo pooing' the idea of asking the patients anyway [GP]

The group's approach to task completion did not appear to adhere to a set timetable. One group member felt a timetable may have assisted the process of task completion.

> I think it would have been useful to have a timetable of events because it did seem to drag on a bit while we went from session to session trying to decide what we were going to do. I think the longer that drags on the less the enthusiasm becomes [GP]

The group commenced with a recognized leader. Owing to unforeseen circumstances, the initial leader had to leave the group and provided a replacement upon her departure, though not from within the group. Both leaders had attained recognition of their role from all group members and the majority of respondents reported the group had good leadership. However, the interviews revealed that both leaders appeared to play the role of 'small group leader' (Scott and Marinker, 1990).

Can you tell me what your role was within the group?

*Well really it was to coordinate, to act as a go-between if you like between all the speci-
alities, not lead or anything like that. [Small group leader]*

Despite not achieving any of the aims it set itself, the group members gained a
great deal from their participation in the project. Many members reported
feeling a sense of satisfaction in being part of an audit at the interface. Most
members appeared to welcome the opportunity to work with practitioners
from other sectors and felt that they had learned from the experience.

*When I first got involved it was just going to be between primary and secondary, but then
it was indicated about the possibility of including social services which was very positive.
I'm sure there's lots of criticisms you could make about how we've actually gone about that
but the sheer fact that we have I think we deserve a star for that [Health and Social Needs
Facilitator]*

*I think I'd be a bit more aware of the holes you can fall into. I think I'd be on the look out for
them, so yes, I think I did gain out of it although I'm not convinced that I'm going to get a
lot of useful information out of the audit so far [GP]*

6.5   IMPLICATIONS FOR IMPLEMENTING CHANGE IN
INTERFACE AUDIT

From the two studies, we have produced two complementary views of the
issues within interface audit. We have produced a detailed picture of aspects
of the structure and process of a sample of audit activity across the primary–
secondary care interface in England and Wales, and we have presented a case
study of an interface audit group that did not complete its audit and subsequently disbanded.

While it is possible to draw out a number of messages for those undertaking or
considering interface audit, in considering these results it is necessary to be
aware of the strengths and weaknesses of the two studies. Within the survey,
we must consider the sampling approach and the representativeness of respondents. The main strength of the cascade sampling approach that we used is in
providing an appropriate sampling frame where no other explicit list of appropriate individuals exists. We did not have, and still do not know of, any comprehensive register of interface audits that we could have used; this made the
cascade approach the only choice. It is also possible that the survey findings
may represent an over-optimistic view of interface audit because audits
regarded by respondents as successful may have been more likely to be
reported. Indeed, the generally positive views elicited by this survey contrast
with the more negative experiences both from the case study and findings
reported elsewhere (Chambers et al, 1996).

The case study involved the experiences of one interface audit group; the findings of such a study cannot be presented as typical or predictive of future interface groups. As Yin (1990) notes: 'case studies, like experiments, are generalizable to theoretical propositions and not to populations or universes. In this sense, the case study does not represent a "sample" and the investigator's goal is to expand and generalize theories (analytic generalization) and not to enumerate frequencies (statistical generalization).' The experiences of the case study group have suggested that, because of their multi-disciplinary membership and large size, interface audit groups may encounter the generic problems of group work. The questionnaire survey highlighted some positive aspects of working with a large group, but also showed that disagreement was more likely to occur in larger groups. Taken together, these findings suggest that particular attention may need to be given to group membership and group dynamics within interface audit groups. While larger groups can enhance certain outcomes (e.g. discussion of issues of common concern), problems with group process (e.g. disagreement, domination by the few) are more common, as evidenced by both the survey and case study and echoing the literature on small group theory (Scott and Marinker, 1990; Firth-Cozens, 1992; see Chapter 7).

Both studies suggest that deciding who are legitimate stakeholders in the task and need to be involved should be explicitly addressed. The survey showed that certain disciplines were rarely involved as active members of the audit group and instead acted mainly in a support role. The case study pointed to people who were being audited without being fully aware of the fact. In addition, since interface audit brings together agencies and professionals who have more traditionally worked apart, there is a theoretical risk that lack of shared knowledge about the aims, goals and role of each participating agency may allow suspicion and mistrust to develop. The issues of trust and shared understanding were highlighted by both studies, with a sense of mistrust being identified as a possible impeding factor in the case study, and the shared understanding resulting from prior knowledge of other group members being identified as contributory factors to successful group working. Therefore, in interface audit, it is particularly important to be aware of the backgrounds and aims of group members who may feel a greater loyalty to the profession they are representing than to a common group goal.

Although within the survey we did not enquire about group leadership, the identified need for effective group working plus the results of the case study support the importance of skilled small group leadership in such groups (Scott and Marinker, 1990; Eccles et al, 1996b). Previous authors have identified a number of important responsibilities of the small group leader (Firth Cozens, 1992; Spencer, 1993). These include: to assign tasks and ensure that the group works on these; to manage conflict; to check on performance and monitor progress against set deadlines.

Lack of a timetable against which progress was monitored was highlighted as a possible contributing factor to group problems in the case study. The group task is an important structural factor influencing any group's success (Krech et al, 1962; Ambulatory Care Programme, 1991). The experience of groups setting standards suggested that the group task should be realistic in terms of all resources available and have the full commitment of all group members (Newton et al, 1992). However, within the case study, establishing a common, achievable group task to which all members were committed was particularly difficult, and trying to achieve this resulted in the group splitting. The majority of respondents to the survey felt their group task was well understood, but highlighted joint initiation of an audit as a facilitating factor. The fact that the audit in the case study was initially the idea of a pre-existing group rather than the interface audit group may have contributed to its problems. Attempts to incorporate a diversity of approaches to, and views about, a topic will run the risk of such splits or of expanding the group task beyond the limits of resources available. The survey results also suggest that time may be a crucial factor in enhancing understanding of the task – allowing sufficient time in meetings for discussion and clarification of objectives is important.

The potential for differences and conflict between members is greater within a multidisciplinary group. If this can be used constructively, difference and conflict is not a weakness but a strength of such groups. As Firth Cozens (1992) observes: 'Groups composed of highly similar individuals who hold common beliefs and have similar abilities are likely to view a task from a single perspective. Although solidarity can be useful it can also lead to an absence of critical thought necessary for evaluating complex problems, and for decision making the gradual process of teasing out the elements of good patient care can be achieved only by including in the team representatives of all those involved in that care'. The extent to which this strength is harnessed and used to its full potential will depend largely on the skills and style of the group leader. It is important that any leader of an interface audit group be aware of the difficult nature of the task they are taking on. In particular, they must be aware of power relationships, and the detrimental effect that these might have on the group process and task achievement. In both the survey and the case study, the dominance of doctors was noted. Without a greater breadth of knowledge of audits, it is difficult to set this in perspective, but it does suggest the scope for greater, and more equitable involvement of other health care professionals. This could be seen as a general message and not specific to interface audit; nonetheless, it is more likely to be an issue at the primary–secondary care interface, since there are more disciplines who are potential participants and who could therefore have a legitimate input. Those who provide an input but are not full and equal members of the group are likely to feel disenfranchised. This lack of involvement is a potential obstacle to implementing any changes suggested and thus to improving the quality of care.

Lack of time is often given as a reason for not being involved in audit (Spencer, 1993; McColl et al, 1994), and doctors view audit as time consuming (Chambers et al, 1996). While lack of time was not highlighted within the case study, respondents to the survey suggested that longer meetings are beneficial in fostering good understanding and allowing for interchange of ideas; this suggests that protected time for audit meetings may be necessary if audit of this kind is to achieve its full potential. Sufficient time was one of the factors identified by respondents as likely to facilitate further interface audits.

Structural obstacles between disciplines and sectors are self-evidently more likely to occur in audits across a divide. Problems of this nature were highlighted by both the survey, which alluded to particular problems with computer incompatibility and geographical distance between members, and the case study, which pinpointed language barriers, lack of shared knowledge and understanding of systems and mismatches of geographical boundaries. Efforts to overcome these obstacles will be necessary in any interface audit activity.

The findings from the survey on progress around the audit cycle are complex to interpret. The 22% of completed audits that had gone through all the steps of the audit cycle, including re-auditing, clearly had the potential to be using audit to improve quality of care. Similarly, just over a quarter of incomplete audits had got as far as implementing change. However, almost two-thirds of audit groups that reported their work as complete had stopped short of implementing change. It has been suggested that failure to close the audit loop means that audit is rendered near useless, and a waste of time and money. Authors have decried the 'failure' of audit to get as far as the remedial action of suggesting and implementing change (Crombie and Davies, 1994; DeDombal, 1994). Our findings quantify for interface audit what Baker (1994) and others have said about this failure. The amount of money already spent on audit has been questioned on the grounds of lack of evidence of effectiveness (Maynard, 1993). The ultimate criterion of audit success has to be improved quality of care. While our findings from both the survey and the case study show it to be an enjoyable educational exercise with the potential to improve communication and professional development, to move interface audit beyond this, future initiatives must emphasize the importance of completing the audit cycle.

Nonetheless, we conclude that interface audit is occurring, is enjoyable and has the scope to improve the quality of care. However, there are issues of group dynamics and organization that should be explicitly addressed. In addition, with the majority of audits stopping short of implementing change, the activity seems currently to be limited in its achievement of this goal. If interface audit is to be effective in improving the quality of care, more information is needed about the specific obstacles to change in this context, and strategies developed to overcome them.

6.6 SUMMARY POINTS

- Aspects of care which cross the interface between primary and secondary NHS sectors may sometimes be improved through clinical audit – interface audit.
- Interface audit requires active involvement from both sides of the interface and so will involve working in small groups.
- A questionnaire survey of members of interface audit groups and a case study of one interface audit group showed:

    Group membership affects the likely success.

    All stakeholders should be represented in the group.

    Dominance by doctors is likely and should be avoided.

    Objectives need to be agreed and clear.

    Conflicts will appear but can be addressed.

    Protected time for meetings is recommended.

    Structural barriers can be identified and solutions or compromises agreed.

    Interface audits are no more likely to complete the audit cycle than audits in other settings.

    Interface audits improve communication between primary and secondary care professionals, encourage professional development and are enjoyable.

ACKNOWLEDGEMENTS

We are grateful to Allen Hutchinson for the initiation of the Interface Audit Project, to Helen Richardson for her work on the project and to the former Northern Regional Health Authority for funding both it and the interview study. We are grateful to the group members for their co-operation with this latter study. We would like to thank the Interface Audit Project steering group of Mr R. Attard, Dr C. Bradshaw, Dr C. Davidson, Dr W. Ennis, Dr A. Hendricks and Dr J. Woodhouse. We also thank Sylvia Hudson for secretarial support in conducting the survey and Zoe Clapp for her input into the conduct of the second phase of the survey.

REFERENCES

Ambulatory Care Programme (1991) *Medical Audit Tools*. Newcastle Upon Tyne: Centre for Health Services Research.

Baker R (1994) What is interface audit? *J R Soc Med* **87**:228–231.

Brown R (1988) *Group Process. Dynamics Within and Between Groups*. Oxford: Blackwell.

Bryce FC, Clayton JK, Rand RJ, Beck I, Farquharson DIM and Jones SE (1990) General practitioner obstetrics in Bradford. *BMJ* **300**:725–727.

Chambers R, Bowyer S and Campbell I (1996) Investigation into the attitudes of general practitioners in Staffordshire to medical audit. *Quality in Health Care* **5**:13–19.

Crombie I and Davies H (1994) What is successful audit? *Managing Audit in General Practice* **2**:6–8.

DeDombal FT (1994) What is wrong with medical audit? *Medical Audit News* **4**:117–120.

Diedrich RC and Dye HA (editors) (1972) *Group Procedures, Purposes, Processes and Outcomes*. Boston: Houghton Mifflin.

Eccles MP, Deverill M, McColl E and Richardson H (1996a) A national survey of audit activity across the primary–secondary interface. *Quality in Health Care* **5**:193–200

Eccles MP, Clapp Z, Grimshaw J, Adams PC, Higgins B, Purves I and Russell I (1996b) Developing valid guidelines: methodological and procedural issues from the North of England evidence based guideline development project. *Quality in Health Care* **5**:44–50.

Firth-Cozens J (1992) Building teams for effective audit. *Quality in Health Care* **1**:252–255.

Irvine D and Irvine S (1991) *Making Sense of Audit*. Oxford: Radcliffe Medical Press.

Krech D, Crutchfield RS and Ballachey EL (1962) *Individual in Society*. New York: McGraw-Hill.

Lawrence M (1993) What is medical audit? In: Lawrence M and Schofield T (editors) *Medical Audit in Primary Care*. Oxford: Oxford University Press.

Levine JM and Moreland R (1990) Progress in small group research. *Annu Rev Psychol* **41**:585–643.

Mantel N and Haenzel W (1959) Statistical aspects of analysis of data from retrospective studies of disease. *J Natl Cancer Inst* **22**:719–748.

Maynard A (1993). Auditing audit. *Medical Audit News* **3**:67–68.

McColl E, Newton J and Hutchinson A (1994) An agenda for change in referral – consensus from general practice. *Br J Gen Pract* **44**:157–162.

Miles B and Huberman AM (1984) *Qualitative Data Analysis. A Source Book of New Methods*. London: Sage.

Newton J, Hutchinson A, Steen N, Russell I and Haimes E (1992) Educational potential of medical audit: observations from a study of small groups setting standards. *Quality in Health Care* **1**:256–259.

Scott M and Marinker ML (1990) Small group work. In: Marinker ML (editor) *Medical Audit and General Practice*. London: BMJ, pp 185–195.

Spencer J (1993) Audit in general practice: where do we go from here? *Quality in Health Care* **2**:183–188.

SPSS Inc. (1990) *SPSS Reference Guide*. Chicago: SPSS Inc.

Yin RK (1990) *Case Study Research. Design and Methods*. California: Sage.

Chapter 7

GOOD CLINICAL AUDIT REQUIRES TEAMWORK

Celia McCrea

7.1 INTRODUCTION

This chapter highlights some of the factors that can lead to obstacles within teams undertaking clinical audit, and suggests a few strategies that can help overcome them. Although teams may have a number of strengths, team conflict and dysfunction may mean that many services are dominated by interprofessional power struggles (Dickens, 1994). It is no use having well considered tactical plans about what to change without a parallel strategy and plans for how to implement them. But, although no one would dream of allowing a student nurse to take a blood sample, or a manager to control a budget, without prior training, many professionals are attempting to undertake multidisciplinary work and clinical audit, unaware of the importance of training to the achievement of effective teamwork.

Beck and Yeager (1996), in discussing problems faced by companies when trying to keep quality initiatives alive, concluded that poor teamwork was one of the biggest causes of failure. Often quality initiatives are typified by employees being sequestered in conference rooms and asked to make use of fishbone diagrams, Pareto charts, histograms, process maps and similar tools. There are timekeepers, gatekeepers, scribes, facilitators and people called leaders, but with no one really leading. When quality teams have the tools to analyse a problem but lack the tools for effective teamwork, the result is often over engineering. The focus becomes the analytical tools; the people and the process end up serving the tools rather than the other way round, and when that happens teams can create elaborate schemes that lead nowhere. For quality initiatives to succeed, people need to be able to work together in teams. But most team leaders receive inadequate training in the fundamentals of how to make a team produce results. They are trained in how to use analysis

Implementing Change With Clinical Audit. Edited by Richard Baker, Hilary Hearnshaw and Noelle Robertson.
© 1999 John Wiley & Sons, Ltd.

and problem solving tools, but not in the leadership skills needed to turn a group of people into a team.

Too often, individual assignments and group efforts are seen as polar opposites, and many trainers even claim 'There are no "I's" or "you's" in the word team'. The implication is that teamwork means involving everyone in a 'we' exercise. This kind of thinking results in the mistaken notion that teamwork only happens when all team members are together in a conference room, whereas in reality not every team requires a carefully orchestrated group effort like that demanded in team sports such as basketball, hockey or football. Some teams, such as golf, tennis and track teams, require individual excellence with limited group interaction. Thus, to lead a successful team effort, team leaders have to know how to capitalize on the group dynamics, and also need to know how to translate group effort into individual accountabilities. Members of the team also need to be trained so that they too can understand group dynamics, and recognize helpful and unhelpful behaviours and attitudes.

In promoting the growth of effective teams, including health care and clinical audit teams, it is useful to consider first the type of team involved. The stage of team development may be a factor in its performance, and therefore a team may need help in moving from one stage to the next. It is essential to build trust within the team, and reduce fear. Individual problem behaviours may also need resolving before the synergy characteristic of effective teams finally emerges. Each of these issues will be discussed in this chapter.

7.2 TYPES OF TEAMS

Johnson and Johnson (1991) describe the typologies of various teams, and how each can be successfully developed. In doing so, they stress that the productivity of teams is not a simple function of team members' technical competencies and task abilities. Although technical superstars can be a great asset, unless all members pursue team success before their own personal ambition, the team will suffer. Therefore, group goals must be set, work patterns structured and practised, the desire for team success built, and a sense of group identity developed.

Using the example of a sales team, Johnson and Johnson (1991) describe three ways that relationships among team members may be structured. (1) In a competitive situation, because bonuses depend on individual sales figures, members of the team will work against each other to be 'the best'. Even if unable to follow up promising leads personally, a team member may not reveal this information to colleagues, because to do so might jeopardize his or her chances of being the top salesperson. (2) If the team works individualistically, each member of the team will strive to meet a personal sales quota. Everyone can succeed or everyone can fail, and the efforts of the sales people are independent. How many sales one person makes has no positive or negative influence on the success of others. (3) When a team is working cooperatively, success depends not only on how many sales one member makes but also on the sales of all the other team members. This means that if one person has more promising leads than he or she can personally follow up, rather than concealing this information, he or she will be motivated to share it with colleagues to increase the overall performance of the team.

From this example, it would appear that teams structured cooperatively will be more productive than teams structured competitively or individualistically. However, the positive results derived from cooperative efforts do not happen automatically, but require careful structuring. For example, positive interdependence should be fostered, and this exists when members of a team realize that they cannot succeed unless the rest of the team do (and *vice versa*), and that they must coordinate their efforts with those of the rest of the team to complete a task, to achieve the overall goal (as opposed to working towards unrelated personal goals). Some strategies for achieving positive interdependence are shown in Box 7.1.

7.3   STAGES OF TEAM GROWTH

Scholtes et al (1994) provide detailed guidance on many strategies and techniques available to assist project teams. In describing Tuckman's model of group

---

Box 7.1   Strategies for achieving positive interdependence

- Goal interdependence (where all members of the team realize that they have a mutual set of goals that everyone is striving to accomplish, and that success depends on all members reaching the goal).
- Reward interdependence (where each member of the group is given the same reward for completing the task, i.e. not just the team member with the highest status).
- Role interdependence (where each member is assigned complementary and interconnected roles).
- Task interdependence (where a division of labour is created so that the actions of one team member have to be completed if the next group member is to complete his or her responsibilities).
- Resumé interdependence (where each member has only a portion of the information, resources, or materials necessary for the task to be completed).

development (1965; Tuckman and Jensen, 1977) (see Box 7.2), these authors liken his first stage of Forming to a group of hesitant swimmers standing by the pool, dabbling their toes in the water. As individuals go through the transition from individual to member status, they are likely to experience a range of feelings, from excitement and optimism, to suspicion, fear and anxiety about the task ahead. During this initial stage little, if anything, will be achieved in terms of project goals due to the fact that a great deal is happening to distract team members' attention.

However, as individuals begin to realize how much work lies ahead, it is normal for them to almost panic. To continue the swimming analogy, Scholtes et al liken this second, Storming stage, to swimmers who have jumped in the water, think they are about to drown, and start thrashing about. Impatient about the lack of progress, and inexperienced about how decisions might best be made, team members will tend to argue about what actions should be taken, and rely solely on their own personal and professional experience rather than collaborate with others. Common behaviours during this stage are likely to include defensiveness and competition; questioning of the wisdom of those who selected the project and appointed other members of the team; the establishment of unrealistic goals, together with concern about work load; and a general tendency towards disunity, tension, jealousy and a perceived pecking order.

As team members get used to working together, Scholtes et al suggest that the swimmers start helping each other to stay afloat rather than competing with one another. Although the many pressures still facing team members mean that in this Norming stage they still have little energy to spend on progressing toward the team's goal, at least they are beginning to understand one another. As differences are worked through, more time and energy are available for the project, and the team is at last able to start making some progress as a sense of team cohesion and harmony replaces competition and conflict.

In the fourth Performing stage, the swimmers demonstrate that they can now swim in concert. Having resolved relationships and expectations, team members begin performing, diagnosing and solving problems, choosing and implementing changes. Suddenly a lot of work can be achieved as the team is now an effective, cohesive unit.

Box 7.2   Tuckman's stages of group development

- Forming.
- Storming.
- Norming.
- Performing.

While suggesting that insight about the typical stages of a team's development should relieve much of the fear members have about the project's success, every team will go through cycles of good and bad times. As the project's progress varies, the team's mood will swing too. Teams will deal with these problems more effectively if they understand and accept the fact that cycles and changes in attitude are normal. Understanding can also encourage a more active approach in terms of learning when and how to avoid or work through group problems.

Tuckman's model was based on a review of literature that was dominated by research with therapy. More recently, some authors have challenged this model of group development. Beck and Yeager (1996), for example, suggest that teams should consider the implications associated with four possible distortions.

Distortion One is the belief that Forming simply means meeting team-mates. In reality, forming requires much more than meeting the other members of the team. It requires clarifying the team's mission, defining goals and roles, and establishing procedures for getting the work done, and the team leader must ensure that these are accomplished. At the outset, a team meets to form around a clear purpose and then focuses on the best ways to accomplish that purpose.

Distortion Two is the assumption that Storming is inevitable. In reality, many teams have become focused and productive without experiencing storms. While storming often occurs, it is not a required stage of group development. Of course, if someone believes it is supposed to happen, that belief can become a self-fulfilling prophecy.

Distortion Three is the belief that when Storming occurs, it eventually turns into Norming by itself. Many team leaders and facilitators are convinced that dwelling on conflicts is the best way to get the team ready to perform. In reality, storms occur because the team is not focused, the mission and goals are ambiguous, the roles are confusing, or the operating principles and procedures are dysfunctional. These problems do not disappear by arguing, or by ignoring them. Focusing a group requires a concerted effort to answer 'What is the team expected to do?' and 'How are the team's efforts going to be coordinated to meet those expectations?'

Distortion Four is the belief that Performing is the end point of a team's development. Teams often go beyond performing to a point at which their performance levels off (or even declines) because they get complacent, start to burn out, get defensive, or try to preserve the *status quo*. These symptoms are likely to arise if teams are put on autopilot once they have hit the performing stage. But if leaders do not assume that performing is the endpoint, they can avoid static or declining performance by refocusing and revitalizing the team's efforts.

7.4 TRUST AND FEAR

Where project teams encounter obstacles from members, a range of causes can usually be predicted, including historic, factual and emotional issues which are not always easy to disentangle. In listing some of the most frequent sources of obstacles to change, Plant (1987) puts fear of the unknown at the top of the list, also highlighting that some obstacles are considerably easier to deal with than others. For example, trust may be the key issue, but it takes considerably longer to rectify mistrust than to correct misinformation or reassure staff about training in new skills.

West (1994) has noted a truism of human behaviour – that commitment and involvement are most likely to occur when people feel safe. People in groups are more likely to take risks in introducing new and improved ways of doing things if they feel they are unlikely to be attacked or denigrated by other group members. An example is the practice nurse who feels that she is being criticized constantly by the general practitioners, and therefore is less likely to suggest new ways of doing things or offer ideas for improving team functioning. West indicates that such a nurse will also be less likely to exercise his or her initiative in improving the quality of health care supplied by the team to the community.

Safety is the affective context within which people are more likely to engage in effective team working based on trust, acceptance, humour, warmth and support. Together, these lead to the involvement, commitment and creativity of team members in team functioning in a positive climate. Although managers may promote these quality principles to health care staff (including gathering data, discussing problems openly, sharing information across specialities, learning quality management lessons from others and fixing the process, not the blame), staff may not always apply them. The obstacles to change stem from a number of factors.

One obstacle to health care quality management is that, compared to most manufacturing or service operations, health care outcomes are difficult to define, measure and control. At the same time, the belief that practitioners control outcomes contributes to a prevailing view that suggests that in the medical world there are no accidents, only physicians and nurses who make mistakes and are therefore incompetent. Such a view leads to a climate of fear and blame, in which health care staff are afraid that their peers will think less of them when outcomes are disappointing.

Deming (1986) has emphasized the need to drive out fear in the workplace, but these fears are deep rooted. Fear stems from the fact that patient outcomes, good or bad, are typically believed to be a function of provider skill alone. In industry, it is accepted that defects can be the result of either common or special causes. In such settings, it is generally accepted that at least 80% of defects are due to management and the system it has created, while fewer than 20% are directly attributable to worker mistakes. In contrast, there is little recognition of the difference between common and special causes in health care. The process is rarely blamed. Even when process issues are investigated, it is generally the practitioner who is put on the line.

Fear often has the effect of causing people to hide information. A possible motive is to protect the professional. Health professionals care deeply about their patients and feel guilty and vulnerable when things go wrong. Also, they may fear that their peers will attack them if information is discussed in public (although such attacks would make sense only if professionals were really in full control and therefore genuinely to blame when things go wrong). Another fear might be that openly discussing problems will increase the risk of malpractice litigation.

7.5 REDUCING FEAR

Achieving high quality health care requires defining high quality care, monitoring practices, and changing the behaviour of practitioners to conform with standards. The obstacle of fear stems from the psychological defences that physicians, nurses and other members of multidisciplinary teams construct. These defences must be addressed before quality improvement can be implemented. Shearer (1996) notes that although it may be fashionable to think that everyone in a successful team is motivated by positive forces such as camaraderie, empowerment, and recognition, in reality these are usually balanced by such factors as fear of rejection, fear of powerlessness, and fear of neglect and isolation.

7.5.1 Defining quality

When fear levels are high, it makes sense to start with steps that do not pose direct threats to individual practitioners. Regular meetings to define processes and outcomes that constitute high quality care provide a non-threatening forum that raises awareness of quality issues. Developing standards also sets the stage for the next important step of gathering and reporting information on current practices.

7.5.2 Monitoring and analysing processes and outcomes

Monitoring performance requires data collection and information dissemination. Again, to minimize the obstacle of resistance to sharing usually confidential information, meetings should be scheduled regularly to provide a forum for discussing general information as well as specific adverse outcomes. Discussion of all cases of adverse outcome can also eliminate the fear of being singled out, and reinforces the notion that common causes for problems exist and can be systematically studied. The key point to establish is that there can be potential for improving performance without the need to label actions as malpractice.

7.5.3   Changing professionals' behaviour

Health professionals need to believe that discussing system problems will actually lead to system improvement. If providers feel that their practice is being supported, they will be more likely to be open about adverse outcomes and look to solutions that might prevent similar outcomes for themselves and others in the future. If problems are identified, they must be addressed.

Exploring ways by which management and teams can focus on eliminating this intangible enemy, Kivenko (1994) notes that fear of failure, fear of supervisors, fear of voicing an opinion, and fear of change, are the chief enemies of timely action and flexibility. Until fear is minimized or eliminated, experimentation with new concepts will not become commonplace.

To reduce fear, one of the main strategies is to open channels for two-way communication (see Chapter 9). Management must be frank and honest, and provide timely information. Managers must not only provide employees with information, they must also provide ways for employees to communicate with them. The potential benefits associated with such strategies are highlighted in the example presented by Crom and France (1996) of a UK company involved in the manufacture of cardboard packaging. The climate in this hierarchical organization was one of fear. Employees were afraid to take risks and each department worked within its own well-established turf. But project teams were then established, and central to the teams' problem-solving approach was the belief that employees have many ideas on how to improve their work processes and would gladly implement those ideas if given sufficient time, training and management support.

During training, teams met with senior management to receive their mission and to hear the declaration of management's commitment and support. Given the employees' past experiences, serious doubts about management's sincerity were voiced. What followed was a healthy, open exchange in which managers challenged the teams to test their sincerity by coming forward with specific requests, and by asking for their support on decisions when needed. This cleared the air and set the stage for moving forward.

Naturally, doubt about management's support persisted among many team members until experience taught them otherwise. Once the teams' initial requests were approved and other types of top management support were demonstrated, doubts subsided and fear was replaced with trust. This desirable outcome was only achieved because, from the outset, the directors recognized that the existing company culture would be an obstacle to employees exercising their initiative and being creative in their problem solving efforts. By attending team meetings and asking team members, 'How can I help?', senior management indicated that the improvement effort was taken seriously and participation in it worthwhile. This example illustrates how teams succeed when they have confidence in themselves, their managers, the training, and the opportunity to make changes in the way work gets done.

Suggesting strategies for addressing ten reasons why people resist participating in teams, Jaycox (1996) highlights the importance of addressing mistrust of management by ensuring open, honest communication between teams, management, and the overall organizational community. While teams respect confidentiality when this is needed, information sharing is also a vital part of team strategy, especially when it can serve to demonstrate that decisions are based on shared values and goals, and that the team has ownership of the process. With such open and honest communication, team members are less likely to be sceptical of the motives of management, and team enthusiasm is more likely to be engendered, even to confirmed pessimists.

However, one caveat should be added in the context of moving from a climate of fear to one of trust. Frequently, well-intentioned efforts to promote trust can become counter-productive, usually due to the mistaken belief that some quick 'team building' exercise will be able to achieve the transition. Instead trust must be earned. While it may take a long period for evidence to build up which leads to a decline in levels of suspicion, one brief incident (such as an action which appears to prove that previous mistrust was justified) can swiftly undermine this effort with mistrust returning to initial or even greater levels.

7.6   DEALING WITH PROBLEM BEHAVIOURS

While teams will invariably face a wide range of problems, it is likely to be individual obstructive behaviours which most interfere with the team's effectiveness. Because many people have never been trained, or required to work as part of a team, they often lack the skills needed. Forsha (1992) argues that personal change is at the heart of all quality activities, and the ways in which we socialize with each other are rooted in our animal nature. An understanding of some of these behaviours can be helpful in working with others in an organization and also building teams. Three of the most common types of behaviours are mounting, grooming and manipulation, and these behaviours may be observed in bosses, peers, or subordinates.

7.6.1 Mounting behaviour

Mounting behaviour is easy to observe in animals but with humans it is shown in more subtle ways. Some animals from time to time will climb up on another's back, the usual purpose of which is to show dominance. The analogous mounting behaviour in humans occurs when one person puts someone down, particularly in the presence of others. If you are the subject of such behaviour, it may be easier to bear when you are aware that the person is trying to express dominance. Back stabbing, backshooting, bullying, gatekeeping and the back burner are examples of mounting behaviour. In each case, one person expresses dominance over another by controlling the situation. A few ways to overcome back stabbing are:

- Encourage up-front communication.
- Avoid stabbing others in the back.
- Use facts to counter unfair accusations.

Backshooting is another manifestation of mounting behaviour in which the outcome can be worse for the attacker than for the victim. It can occur when a decision needs to be made but your associate does not want to take the risk of being wrong, so he or she delays until you must make the decision. If it turns out to be wrong, you are criticized. The best defence is to get input from the other interested parties before making a final decision. The irony of this example is that it eventually forces all decisions onto the backshooter as other people become aware of the game and refuse to play. As a result, this person frequently feels overwhelmed by all the work.

Bullying is one of the oldest tricks in the book, and is usually perpetrated by someone who is insecure. Knowing this does not help you deal with the bully's behaviour, but it helps to understand that he or she is compensating for perceived weaknesses. The way to handle a bully may be assumed to be just as rough, but it can be more helpful to let bullies blow off steam then ask what you can do to help.

Another way to seek dominance is by gatekeeping or channelling. Gatekeeping is a normal part of the working chain of command, with information being passed up and down the chain and issues being handled at the appropriate level. It is a way to control information and action, but it becomes maladaptive when someone avoids notifying your of changes that affect your job, acts as an intermediary between you and your supervisors and associates, or provides indirect feedback on situations in which you are directly involved. It may not be possible to eliminate gatekeeping, but it can be controlled through being aware of its use and substituting first-hand conversation and your best judgement for hearsay and innuendo (Forsha, 1992).

Just because something is important to you does not mean that it is important to somebody else. Many actions require the coordinated efforts of several people. If one person puts a project on the back burner, he or she can hold up the whole process. This constitutes mounting behaviour in that by controlling the situation, the individual puts him/herself in a position of dominance. One solution is to instigate a series of regular prompts, so that after a certain amount of follow-up, the person who is dragging his or her feet will get going. But in this context, it is important to remember that more bees are caught with honey than with vinegar. Gentle persistence is the watchword. Confrontation should be saved for the times when it is absolutely necessary.

7.6.2 Grooming

Grooming behaviour is the opposite of mounting. By grooming somebody you are extending friendship, warmth and cooperation. Grooming behaviour is an essential part of any relationship, for example, the compliment. In the day-to-day world of making things happen, it is easy to forget to compliment others. Good managers or team leaders remember to praise freely, but the praise must be sincere. It takes a continuous flow of grooming to create an atmosphere that will reduce the stresses of daily work, and unfortunately one negative comment can wipe out a lot of goodwill.

Consideration and integrity are other facets of grooming. We do not always agree with one another, but it is particularly frustrating when you think the other person is not listening to your point of view. Therefore, it is important to give full consideration to the other person's thoughts and feelings before taking action. This requires discipline and time, but listening to others helps improve your decisions as well as working relationships.

In all team work where grooming is used, a final ingredient is integrity. You are honest in issues and respectfully agree, or disagree or side-step an issue without confusing your associates. A lack of integrity leaves colleagues continually doubting your motives.

7.6.3 Manipulation

This is the third type of individual problem behaviour commonly seen in organizations. Manipulation occurs when we trick people into doing something. The manipulator does something that is in his or her best interest while pretending to help others. People eventually see this for exactly what it is.

Some of the most common forms of manipulation relate to the rage reaction. The rage reaction might be what the bull feels when it charges. Every now and then, someone who is typically easy-going and even-tempered sees red. Then watch out. Eventually this will pass and the person will probably feel some remorse. It is important to distinguish between this instant, off-guard rage response and other forms of anger. The former usually means you have hit a sensitive spot. Now you have some good information you can use it constructively. Later, when the person is more relaxed, you can take your time and discuss in a non-threatening way what it was that made him or her mad. But if the rage occurs frequently or if the rage is extreme, we are not dealing with a quality improvement problem and we should not offer a quality improvement solution. When someone is not in control of his or her emotions, you are better off picking another time to discuss your quality improvement suggestions.

Basing actions on assumption is ineffective and frequently leads to wasted time and effort. It is not always deliberate, but when it is, it is manipulative behaviour. An agenda is simply a list of the actions you have planned. A hidden agenda is what you really want but do not disclose. Unless you are an outstanding manipulator, the hidden agenda will eventually be discovered and you will be discredited. You can spot someone who is using a hidden agenda because his or her actions do not make sense. Once you discover the real agenda, everything falls into place.

Lip service is happening when somebody supports your idea on the surface, compliments it in public, but quietly refuses to take any action to support it. It is among the most frustrating things somebody can do. It is a stupendous waste of time to support with words what you have no intention of carrying out with actions. Why do it?

7.7 CONCLUSION

Effective teamwork requires effective leadership. This should enable the team to overcome obstacles it may encounter in proceeding through stages of development and achieving a cooperative style. Team leaders should also understand problem behaviours as forms of communication and use strategies to resolve them.

Since both health care and clinical audit depend on the quality of teamwork, more attention needs to be given to the development of appropriate skills of team leadership. Box 7.3 provides an example, drawing on the hypothetical case study used in Chapter 4.

Box 7.3   Improving teamwork hypothetical case study

The case study used in Chapter 4 concerned an audit undertaken by an Accident and Emergency Department to improve the use of thrombolytic therapy in patients with acute myocardial infarction. Suppose Dr Wilson, who led the audit, noted that the main obstacle to change was poor teamwork. She sought advice about how to address the problem from a manager, who suggested that since she was the leader of the team it might help if she were to develop her team leadership skills.

Dr Wilson did some reading and attended a short course, then decided to put what she had learnt into practice. From what she had learnt, it seemed likely that her team had not reached the Norming stage, and had yet to establish a clear purpose. She also thought that grooming behaviours such as praise were uncommon in the team, although criticisms were expressed more freely, and she suspected there might be an element of fear among team members that cases they had managed individually and omitted thrombolytic treatment might be discussed.

In order to begin to focus the team, she circulated a detailed agenda before the next meeting. At that meeting, she reminded the team about their rules of confidentiality as well as the objectives they had agreed for the audit of the use of thrombolytics. Then she told them about a case she had managed in which she had failed to administer thrombolytic treatment in the Accident and Emergency Department. She asked the group to use their own similar experiences to identify reasons why they omitted to use thrombolytic treatment. During the subsequent discussion, she was careful to discourage critical comments between members of the team, and used compliments when appropriate.

Dr Wilson accepted that it would take time to establish trust and enable the team to work in a different way. By the end of the meeting, most team members had been able to report occasions when thrombolytics might have been used but were not, although some still appeared to be reluctant to discuss the issue. However, over a few meetings everyone began to take a full part. They also made suggestions about how to improve performance, and set aside a meeting to identify the obstacles to change in more detail.

In the meetings that followed, the team gradually developed a more cooperative method of working. They identified several obstacles to change, most of which they were able to overcome, and the findings of the next data collection 18 months later confirmed that performance had improved considerably. Dr Wilson was surprised at how long the process had taken, but also noted that there had been other benefits from the improved team work.

7.8 SUMMARY POINTS

- Good clinical audit requires teamwork.
- Obstacles can occur within teams, but there are strategies which can help to overcome them.
- Team members can work as competitors, as individuals or in cooperation.
- Teams can be helped in dealing with the stages of Forming, Storming, Norming and Performing.
- Commitment to the team is higher when team members feel safe rather than when they are fearful.
- There are well described ways to reduce potential fears.
- Team members can behave as obstructive individuals but such behaviours can be prevented or dealt with.

REFERENCES

Beck JDW and Yeager NM (1996) How to prevent teams from failing. *Quality Progress* **29**:27–31.

Crom S and France H (1996) Teamwork brings breakthrough improvements in quality and climate. *Quality Progress* **29**:39–42.

Deming WE (1986) *Out of the Crisis.* Cambridge, Mass.: MIT Center for Advanced Engineering Study.

Dickens P (1994) *Quality and Excellence in Human Services.* Chichester: Wiley Series in Clinical Psychology.

Forsha HI (1992) The pursuit of quality through personal change. *Quality Progress* **29**:110–113.

Jaycox M (1996) How to get non-believers to participate in teams. *Quality Progress* **29**:45–49.

Johnson DW and Johnson FP (1991) *Joining Together: Group Theory and Group Skills.* Fourth edition. London: Prentice-Hall International Editions.

Kivenko K (1994) Improve performance by driving out fear. *Quality Progress* **27**:1994.

Plant R (1987) *Managing Change and Making it Stick.* London: Gower.

Scholtes PR, Bayless DL, Massaro GL and Roche NK (1994) *The Team Handbook – How to Use Teams to Improve Quality.* Madison, WI: Joiner Associates, Inc.

Shearer C (1996) TQM requires the harnessing of fear. *Quality Progress* **29**:97–100.

Tuckman BW (1965) Development sequence in small groups. *Psychological Bulletin* **63**:384–399.

Tuckman BW and Jensen MA (1977) Stages of small group development revisited. *Group and Organisational Studies* **2**:411–427.

West M (1994) *Effective Teamwork.* London: British Psychological Society.

Chapter 8

IMPLEMENTING CHANGE WITH AUDIT: THE ROLE OF MANAGEMENT

Jonathan Shapiro

8.1 INTRODUCTION

Although the concept of auditing health services is hardly new (we only need to look at Florence Nightingale, measuring survival rates before and after the introduction of antisepsis in the early nineteenth century), the concept of integrating financial and clinical audit effectively in order to manage health care is one which has only arisen over the past few years. In this chapter, we shall look at the emergence of managerially led audit, review the manner in which non-clinical and clinical audit have begun to integrate, and consider options for the future.

Within the NHS, audit generally seems to have entered the culture by means of a pincer movement from two different directions. On the one hand, there has been the financially driven, process orientated, traditional form of audit, whilst on the other hand has been clinically driven audit with its strong sense of values and weaker sense of pragmatism.

Both approaches are characterized by strong, somewhat derogatory stereotypes; financially driven audit is traditionally carried out by 'grey suited bureaucrats' driven only by 'the bottom line', who are unable or unwilling to consider any of the softer issues of medicine which are not amenable to ready measurement. Clinical audit by comparison has been seen to be professionally driven by those who are more concerned with clinical care than with cash, whose altruism is outweighed only by their scientific precision and their desire to achieve best practice. Thus, hospital consultants are seen as the most pure

Implementing Change With Clinical Audit. Edited by Richard Baker, Hilary Hearnshaw and Noelle Robertson.
© 1999 John Wiley & Sons, Ltd.

exponents of clinical audit, but administrators are seen to be fit for nothing more than totting up balance sheets.

The value judgements are plain to see, and the difficulties of bringing together the two forms of audit easy to understand. With these judgements comes mutual distrust, which lies even deeper in the roots of society, a distrust which relates to the concept of professionalism.

8.2   PROFESSIONALISM

The professions, whether medical, legal, or financial, are based on the triple pillars of self-selection, monopoly, and self-regulation, all values which were at their peak at the end of the nineteenth century. The medical royal colleges epitomize this concept, with their closed shop approach to the selection of members (physicians, surgeons, and now even nurses and general practitioners), permission to practice being controlled by the attainment of such membership. The General Medical Council's iron grip on judging professional misconduct also emphasizes this point. Anyone who has not passed through these rites of passage is *de facto* not a professional, and hence not seen to be worthy of respect or consideration.

In contrast, particularly in the early days of the NHS when the value systems first became ingrained, administrators often worked their way up the bureaucratic ladder, developing their skills and prejudices in a long apprenticeship which threw them into contact with the worst of clinical practice, and gave them a view of professionals which was entirely at odds with the public perception. Thus, administrators spent the majority of their efforts policing the poorly performing clinicians, rather than developing leading edge clinical practice. They understood how to restrict and control, but were less experienced at enhancing and empowering. The game was played around rules and regulations, with the implication of checking and counting; as we shall see, this merely deepened the rift in thinking between the apparently patient focused clinicians and their seemingly pedantic administrative support.

As the NHS has grown, and society more generally has changed, so these emphases have also subtly altered. We no longer accept the authority of the professional as trustingly as we once did; we want to know the 'why' as well as the 'what', whether in the garage when our cars are being serviced, or when our accountants are held overtly responsible for their opinions, or when we sue our teachers for using the wrong teaching style. So society's clinical practitioners are expected to be more accountable, and management is seen as having a role in acting as the people's champion against the omnipotent professions. This is clearly not the right climate to develop an educational shared approach to audit; is there any way in which such a cultural chasm may be bridged, and the different forms of audit integrated and made consistent?

8.3   A SHARED APPROACH TO AUDIT – BRIDGING THE GAP

8.3.1   Early developments

For answer, we need to look at the development of audit along each of the pathways already described. Since clinical audit has featured so largely in other parts of this book, the emphasis in this chapter will be on the development of management within the NHS, the values that underlie it, and the manner in which it may contribute to effective, efficient care.

When the NHS was created in the late 1940s, its key attributes were intended to be the seamlessness of its networks across the country, and the quality of care which could be delivered to all patients, irrespective of their geography, demography or income. The rise of the district general hospital that offered the same services in every part of the country, and the ideas of equality as much as equity, were both central to the atmosphere of societal altruism which prevailed at that time. In the post-war welfare state mentality which then prevailed, such a system was inevitably very centrally driven, and largely controlled by regulation rather than management.

Thus, NHS institutions were paid for *being* rather than for *doing*, and all expenditure, from vast capital projects down to the provision of hospital meals, was determined centrally. Hospitals were allocated a budget each year, but what services were provided for the money was not clearly identified. General practitioners were paid by their list size, and by a few items of service, but there was no easy way of checking on what they actually did. Those staff not involved in direct patient care worked as administrators with very limited discretionary powers. In essence, they monitored processes and ensured that they conformed to the regulations. During these times, the NHS was 'under-scrutinized and over-regulated' in the sense that processes were monitored but outcomes were not. Funds were largely non-cash limited (that is, there was no formal limit, and there was enough money to cover all the calls on it), so there was little pressure to do more than regulate their use.

In such a system, the origins of managerial audit can easily be detected; process was all important, and the content of activity was left largely untouched. Such an approach appeared to work, as long as there were sufficient resources to run the NHS and prioritizing decisions was not required. Until the mid-1980s, activity within the NHS grew at a rate which was largely acceptable to its political masters, and the government was prepared to resource this predictable rate of growth. However, as improvements in clinical technology grew apace, it became evident that the NHS was likely to absorb resources above and beyond those which were being allocated.

New machines appeared too rapidly to warrant the replacement of old ones, new drugs were able to treat conditions which had previously been incurable, and covert prioritization began to be a feature of the service: waiting lists lengthened and pressure for extra funding began to grow. This meant that for the first time, real choices were required between what should be done and what could be done. Administrators, with their background in regulation and their focus on process, were no longer able to control the service.

At the same time, awareness grew amongst those who finance the NHS that much of its discretionary activity was governed by clinicians. New services appeared when hospital consultants expressed an interest in them; a service would be opened, and patients would be referred. Waiting lists lengthened in those disease areas where clinicians had less interest, or where demand rose more quickly than supply of service; and in the community, the quality of provision of general practice was by and large governed by the whim and enthusiasm of local general practitioners. The provision of services was being determined on an arbitrary, fragmented basis by clinicians in general and doctors in particular.

The system had thus developed two mutually reinforcing weaknesses: resources were no longer able to match the demands placed upon them, and at the same time administrators lost their effectiveness, and clinicians thus gained in influence. A dangerous positive feedback loop was being created at precisely the time when tighter control of the system was required. In response to this state of affairs, the concept of general management was introduced by the Conservative government in 1985, following the publication of the Griffiths report (NHS Management Inquiry, 1983) which recommended tighter managerial control of the NHS. The Griffiths report suggested that running the NHS was like running any other large organization, and that the management skills required were the same, and this *credo* began to be put into practice. In hospitals, management hierarchies began to be formed, and a fairly directive style of leadership emerged, which initially alienated consultants, but which eventually persuaded at least some of them to come on board, if only because they felt that they could do it better. Clinical directorates developed, their focus primarily on activity and efficiency, although the notion of clinical audit followed fairly quickly.

When hospital general management failed to contain the growth of the service, and the crisis in waiting lists became politically unacceptable, the Government followed up on their earlier ideas by introducing the purchaser/provider split and the internal market in health care (Secretary of State, 1990). What do these concepts mean, and what was the relevance of audit to them?

The introduction of general management marked the demise of the NHS administrator, who was to be replaced by the NHS manager. As in the hospitals, so by 1990 these changes had also been introduced in the Family Practitioner Committees which then became Family Health Services Authorities, with all their implications of strength. Where the former had no discretionary power and were required always to follow rules, the latter were given varying amounts of discretion over the way in which public funds were disbursed, and an increasing freedom from tight, centralized rule making.

Thus, where previously non-cash limited funds for general practitioners' premises were made available on the basis of room sizes and car parking spaces, now a cash limited sum was available for those practices which could demonstrate a specific need for new or improved premises. Moreover, they had to show that their needs were greater than those of the neighbouring practices. The judgements were made by managers, and often on the basis of criteria which were not obvious or explicit. Similarly in the hospital sector, clinical directorates which had previously been able to develop their own individual initiatives found themselves vying with each other for limited resources with which to develop new services. Clinician initiative began to be curtailed and the options for innovation to look more limited.

There was a certain irony in all these events, since the reality of service change was driven less by purchasers' decisions than by the rising tide of activity and public demand. The NHS efficiency index of the time rewarded those providers whose activities had gone up most for the least growth in expenditure. This encouraged hospitals merely to do more and more, rather than looking at the health benefits of their activities; emergency admissions, for example, were rising by an average of 5 or 6% annually, for no very clear reason. Despite all the rhetoric about managerial control of the system, each year ended with most hospital trusts (certainly in the acute sector) carrying out many more procedures than they had been contracted to do, and left them effectively underfunded.

Put more plainly, every time contracts were let with hospital trusts to provide services, demand for those services exceeded expectation, and so created *de facto* prioritization in favour of acute conditions and against more elective activity. People with cancer or broken limbs were treated, but those waiting for hip replacements or coronary artery bypass grafts had to wait ever longer.

8.3.2   The introduction of clinical audit

All this while, audit amongst clinicians was being encouraged both within the medical profession and from the outside. At a primary care level, the introduction of medical audit advisory groups (MAAGs) put the onus of responsibility onto primary health care teams to take part in some audit activity. Similarly, hospital consultants were encouraged to carry out audit work; in their case, they had protected time for audit, and were given assistance in the form of information technology and audit staff to help them in these activities. Both in hospitals and in the community, the choice of audit topics was left largely to the clinicians concerned, and much care was taken to ensure that clinician confidentiality was preserved.

Such freedom was seen as a necessary part of the development of audit, in that it was hoped that an appeal to the professional side of a clinician's mindset would encourage audit to be carried out for the 'right' reasons rather than out of necessity or for financial gain. Many of the early audits carried out by MAAGs, for example, were used to demonstrate the benefit of change and the lack of threat, rather than to have any great influence on the delivery of care. The Leicestershire vitamin B_{12} project was carefully chosen to illustrate the ease and benefit of carrying out a large scale audit, rather than to have a dramatic effect on the costs or standards of care, and it certainly succeeded in recruiting most of the local general practitioners into the process, and in consequence helped them to gain a better understanding of audit mechanisms (Fraser et al, 1995).

In places where management was immature, managers did not really appreciate this developmental approach, and tried to drive the clinical audit agenda too early and too quickly. They insisted that valuable NHS resources had to be used only for meaningful audit. In these cases, meaningful was defined in managerial terms, without understanding that definitions of meaning and relevance were highly dependent on perspective and particular interests.

Where the management agenda was imposed on the clinical one, clinicians, like all good professionals, simply played the system and subverted the agenda to their own ends. A lot of public money was used in ineffective activity, whose statistics and outcomes could rarely be believed, let alone trusted. Where management in health authorities was more mature, there was an awareness that the integration of clinical audit with the managerial process would take time, and that it had to be seen to be led by the clinicians in order to maintain their self-respect, ownership and commitment. Whilst such aspirations may sound grandiose and irrelevant in a modern health service, the realities of any professionally led service are that the motivation of clinicians can make or break the system.

I have suggested that unmotivated clinicians play the system; conversely, clinicians who feel involved and understand the value of their activities are much more likely to apply the system for maximum effect and benefit. The introduction of health promotion clinics in the early 1990s was an excellent example of the former, with practices driving activity up to enormous levels of expenditure by performing activities in which they had no faith whatsoever. When clinicians valued the initiatives, as in the more recent chronic disease management programmes, their activity was more measured, and less exploitative.

Where managers understood this, they spent considerable time and effort in enhancing clinicians' sense of involvement. In these cases, audit groups in primary and secondary care were allowed their autonomy for some years, health authorities refrained from making funding conditional on results, and the early audits were encouraged to be educational in nature rather than service orientated. In these cases, it did not take long for clinicians to hone and refine their audit tools, and offer their newly sharpened instruments of audit to the health authority or trust for use in mutually beneficial projects. Audit groups began to approach the health authorities with ideas for future audits, with the results of existing audits, or in the hope of stimulating discussion which might shape their activity.

Having a selection of locally influential clinicians on the audit groups who were able to work with their clinical colleagues in trust or practices, as well as with the health authority, established a vehicle which had the ability to gather audit information, share the findings with the major purchaser of services, and then work together with the purchaser to reshape provision of the service being reviewed. Once reshaped, there was a greater potential for positive implementation of the changed service if the clinicians who had done the original work were involved; thus new protocols for the treatment of asthma or diabetes, for the management of chest infections or the appropriate referral of people with hernias could all be jointly developed, disseminated and implemented.

And by extension, it began to be seen that having different groupings of clinicians working together would also reap greater benefits; consultants and general practitioners were already beginning to work across the interface between primary and secondary care (see Chapter 6), but others, particularly nurses, now began to join the audit groups.

Apart from the traditional professional drive for clinicians to take part in audit, there was a dawning awareness amongst both clinicians and managers that audit could be used to demonstrate the need for enhanced services, or to reduce ineffective activities and release some resources for other clinical work. Hard pressed hospital directorates began to use audit to highlight the need for more resources; managers would collude with clinicians in using audit to show their straitened circumstances; and directorates of public health medicine were able to point to areas of need by the use of clinical audit.

Where management has been weaker, and the administrative need for process based results has been stronger, there has been an earlier insistence on developing audits which matched the management agenda. Not only were these often inappropriate, in that they concentrated too much on the process of audit and not enough on its outcome, but they also ensured that clinicians felt over-managed and undervalued so that many were tempted to 'work to rule' in their approach to patient services and management involvement.

8.3.3   The future relationship between audit and management

I have described how administrators have evolved into managers, and gained some insight into the manner in which procedurally driven audit could evolve into a potentially powerful management tool in the form of collaborative out-come based audit. This shows that audit is not an incidental addition to health care, but a natural development which has the potential to bridge the divide between clinical and service management.

I have also briefly discussed the manner in which clinicians were involved in the audit process. It does not take a large leap of the imagination to postulate the next step, when managers and clinicians begin to find their roles and functions overlapping and the distinctions between them beginning to blur. Clinical directorates in hospitals have traditionally been led by consultants working with business managers at their right hand, whilst clinical audit in primary care has found multi-disciplinary audit groups [including general practitioners, public health doctors, health authority managers, clinicians from non-medical specialities, support staff, and (in some cases) user groups] working together in loose alliances which promote mutual interdisciplinary respect and trust. If these moves are extrapolated, then one can begin to see the emergence of the hybrid clinical manager, the multi-skilled managerial clinician, or perhaps the new clinical governors.

As in many of the scenarios we have already described, such beings can develop along more than one evolutionary pathway. At their worst, managerial clinicians develop all the characteristics of the old health service administrators. Pedantic to a fault, inflexible, and unimaginative, such beings insist that each number is crunched, each clinical activity measured, and anything that is unquantifiable is ignored. Looking at some of the commercial health mainte-nance organizations from the USA, one can see many of these features coming to life in a terrifying manner. Every clinical activity must be related to its protocol, each prescription must be authorized, and every intervention must have a measurable outcome; the result is technocratic, bureaucratic, reduction-ist medicine which treats human beings like machines, and takes no account of the multi-factorial nature of disease, of human nature, and of successful med-ical intervention. The journey from an over-regulated, under-scrutinized service reaches its apogee by becoming under-regulated and over-scrutinized, a service run by technicians, not by professionals, where discretion and flexibility are dirty words.

However, where the integration has gone well, then powerful, humane and enlightened individuals have emerged who are able to integrate the need for financial viability, technical intervention and human frailty which constitutes the core of good clinical practice. Often, such people have started from a clinical (although not necessarily a medical) background. There are examples here of the part which consultants in public health medicine may have to play, although clinicians from all fields of clinical care have made the transition.

Consultants in public health medicine have the skills in epidemiology and large populations which are needed to develop broad policies from audit work, and indeed, may well be able to help in audit design and implementation. They also have a degree of clinical experience and a knowledge of the managerial environment, and so should be well placed to take on this role between clinical medicine and management. Most audit groups include such consultants in their number, in the same way that an increasing number of health authorities see public health doctors entering senior management.

However, the specific backgrounds of such individuals matter less than their generic characteristics; they must have credibility with their consultants (hence the usefulness, but not the necessity, of a clinical background), they must be flexible and developmental in their approach, and they must have the ability to inspire confidence and the suspension of cynical disbelief among those whom they lead.

For what we are seeing is the need for strong leadership, the need for individuals who have the skills of change management and human resource development, who can kick start the process and create real culture change. Those who are able to commence the process may not be the same as those who complete it; the more successful organizations (whether health authorities, trusts or general practices) are harnessing their leaders, and moving their innovators onto pastures new once the processes of change have been started.

Increasingly, well trained professional managers are appearing who are able to work seamlessly with clinical professionals to gain the same broad view of the care their patients require. With experience in managing large organizations, and the human resource management skills which are not part of most clinicians' basic training, they offer a resource to the system which clinicians on the whole are unequipped or unprepared to provide.

Combining the managerial and clinical skills of both clinicians and managers, with less regard for the traditional professional barriers, offers the opportunity to develop a service which is prepared to be reflective, and questions its values and its practitioners, but is able to do so in a manner which does not threaten its professionals, but merely encourages them to look for improvement and development on a continuing basis. Organizations led by such individuals are self-driven, and are motivated to do their best for patient, for organization, and for the wider population. They are able to ignore structural vested interests, and to focus their activity and those of their organization on the needs of their users.

Such organizations may be focused around health authorities, but they are increasingly also to be seen at smaller population sizes; provider organizations, whether primary care groups, multifunds, or trusts, are all developing this same multi-skilled, multidisciplinary approach, and this is clearly the direction for the future. Audits carried out on appropriate population groupings bring together all the concepts we have mentioned, of appropriateness, professional ownership, and local relevance. For such organizations, audit becomes a self-evidently effective tool, and one that is already becoming recognized. For them, audit is an instrument for encouraging change and developing practice, rather than a lever of power and control.

It remains to be seen whether the introduction of new national organizations in the UK such as the National Institute of Clinical Excellence (NICE) or the Commission for Health Improvement (CHI) mooted in the Labour administration's recent policy document (Secretary of State, 1997) will follow the same precepts. At present, the messages about their *modus operandi* are mixed: NICE seems to be intended to be facilitative and constructive in nature, allowing NHS professionals of all descriptions to have access to the results of studies on effectiveness, and of audits on benefit and best practice.

CHI, on the other hand, seems more likely to represent the stick to NICE's carrot, able to monitor and police poor performance in a manner which may end up both parental and counterproductive unless it is kept in reserve and only used as an ultimate deterrent.

Much of the detail about these organizations has yet to be developed and solidified; their approach may well reflect the manner in which the NHS reacts to the ideas on audit and reflective practice which are contained in the policy document. With a good response, the spiral of positive reinforcement will have been strengthened, and the professionally driven mode of development described in this chapter will move forward; if the service reacts too cynically, or the financial constraints make restriction the order of the day, then the disempowering central mechanisms are more likely to be invoked, and the 'dumbing-down' of the NHS will have moved one step closer. Only time and the attitudes of all those involved in delivery of the service will tell.

8.4   SUMMARY POINTS

- As health care has become more complex, and costs have escalated, systems of health service administration have been replaced by more proactive general management, which seek to play a greater role in the management of clinical care.

- Clinical audit has been introduced to enable health professionals to manage aspects of the quality of care.
- Policies adopted by managers have influenced the effectiveness of audit. When more enlightened approaches have been adopted, more open relationships between professionals and managers have developed, and audit has been of wider use to the health service.
- In the future, a closer, more effective relationship between clinical audit and management is needed. This might be achieved by the emergence of the multi-skilled managerial clinician (perhaps clinical governors). Given leadership abilities and the support of their own organizations and the new national agencies (for example, NICE), they would bring about the culture change that would promote change and continuing improvement in clinical care.

REFERENCES

Fraser RC, Farooqi A and L Sorrie R (1995) Use of vitamin B-12 in Leicestershire practices: single topic audit led by a medical audit advisory group. *BMJ* **311**:28–30.
NHS Management Inquiry (1983) *The Griffiths Report*. London: DHSS.
Secretary of State for Health (1990) *Working For Patients*. London: HMSO.
Secretary of State for Health (1997) *The New NHS. Modern Dependable*. London: HMSO.

Chapter 9

INTERNAL COMMUNICATIONS AND THE MANAGEMENT OF CHANGE

Owen Hargie and Dennis Tourish

9.1 INTRODUCTION

This chapter will focus upon the specific communication implications which impinge upon organizations and the people in them at times of innovation and change. A smooth flow of communication is essential to the success of all organizations. However, during periods of change the need for rapid, open and effective communication is paramount. At such junctures people experience an increased need for uncertainty reduction. If this uncertainty is reduced, then the resulting outcome will be positive, whereas if existing fears and apprehensions are ignored or rejected, the consequence will be organizational dysfunction (Tourish and Hargie, 1993). There is now considerable research to indicate that in times of difficulty, those organizations which pay careful attention to communication by management perform more successfully on a range of criteria than do those in which such communication is poor.

The chapter begins with a review of the role of communication in determining organizational success. The concepts of innovation and change will be delineated, and the communication implications of both highlighted. The nature and results of recent audits of communication in the NHS are then summarized. Finally, the defining characteristics of a communication strategy which enable organizations to deal successfully with change will be emphasized. Throughout the chapter, the interpersonal skills and strategies which have been shown to improve managerial communicative performance will be highlighted.

Implementing Change With Clinical Audit. Edited by Richard Baker, Hilary Hearnshaw and Noelle Robertson.

9.2   COMMUNICATION AND ORGANIZATIONAL SUCCESS

There is a growing body of evidence to support the view that organizational success requires a carefully structured, free flowing system of communication between management and staff (Albrow, 1992). In order to achieve managerial objectives, staff at all levels need to be fully apprised about key issues affecting the organization. Yet many managers seem reluctant to investigate internal communications, are unaware of the role of communication in organizational performance, and do not have a coherent communications strategy (Smith, 1991). Given an already heavy managerial agenda, there may be a reluctance to implement change, since this can mean becoming involved in what may be a difficult process.

While such an attitude is understandable, it is counterproductive. There is now clear evidence that effective internal communications have positive benefits and are an important pre-requisite for the achievement of long-term corporate success. For example, Hanson (1986) found that the presence of good interpersonal relationships between managers and staff was three times more powerful in predicting profitability in 40 major companies over a 5-year period than the four next most powerful variables combined – market share, capital intensity, firm size and sales growth rate. In a comprehensive review of relevant research, Clampitt and Downs (1993) concluded that the outcomes which accrue from good internal communications include increases in quantity and quality of productivity, a decrease in absenteeism, fewer strikes, reduced costs, and greater levels of innovation.

The recent impetus towards organizational restructuring underscores the need for the development of an overall communication strategy. For example, an integral component of the concept of re-engineering is the creation of cross-functional organizational teams each with a multi-purpose remit (Grint, 1994). Where such teams achieve internal cohesion they also generate facilitative intragroup communications, tend to be productive, and engender high member satisfaction (Hargie et al, 1994a). A danger, however, is that such team members can then identify more closely with the team than the organization itself (Barker and Tompkins, 1994). Indeed, this is evident in the NHS where professional staff often identify primarily with their professional colleagues and have a lower sense of identification with the trust or organization to which they belong (Dickson et al, 1997).

This highlights a paradox in the management role, where, on the one hand, the pursuit of effectiveness suggests that employees should work in self-managed teams, while, on the other, a broader organizational loyalty is also a desired objective. A problem is that the formation of teams may lead to distinctive team cultures and loyalties, with their own agenda which may not always be in tandem with overall organizational goals. However, if team development is constrained, then staff empowerment and the delegation of operational tasks become difficult. Overcoming this dilemma may always be a difficult problem, but it will certainly be eased in those organizations where attention is paid to internal communications. As noted by Church (1994, p. 19) 'when systems of communication begin to deteriorate within a given organization, the likelihood increases that the collective set of individuals will fragment into subgroups whose structures reflect their own internal communication needs and dynamics, rather than those of the total organization'. This is particularly the case in those organizations undergoing change, and it is to this issue that we now turn.

9.3 INNOVATION AND CHANGE

Organizational effectiveness increasingly depends to a very large extent on the successful management of both innovation and change (Slappendel, 1996). These two terms are frequently employed as synonyms, with little consideration of the differences between them. In addition, their communication consequences for organizations are often neglected. It is therefore useful to consider the distinction between innovation and change and the communication challenges inherent in both.

While all innovation involves change, not all change involves innovation. Thus, unintended or undesired change would not be innovative. Likewise, many organizational changes are the inevitable adjustments to forced internal or external environmental conditions and pressures. By contrast, an organizational innovation has been defined as: 'an idea, object, or practice perceived as new by an individual or an organization, which is intended to bring about improvement in relation to desired objectives' (Hargie and Tourish, 1996a, p. 4). Thus, innovation involves conscious, planned and directed organizational change.

Innovations can be relatively simple or highly complex. New and different ideas, processes, products or procedures are all examples of innovations. An innovation can take the form of a new system, device, policy, programme, or service and can impact upon all parts of the organization and all aspects of its operation. A review of literature in this field (e.g. Drucker, 1985; West and Farr, 1990; Walker and Henry, 1991; King and Anderson, 1995) highlights the following main features of an innovation:

- It necessitates change.
- It is novel and fundamental in nature.
- It is intentional and planned.
- It can be readily applied.
- It is seen as beneficial.

The process of innovation can be treated either as a single stage or as a longer-term, ongoing, process. The former concentrates largely on simply handling the introduction of the innovation, whereas the latter emphasizes the management of its longer term implementation, including how commitment to the success of the innovation is obtained within the organization. The latter approach is crucial to success. In this perspective, in which innovatory change is viewed as a social process, the interaction between individuals and groups within organizations is seen as a key part of change management, and communication is an essential component of the process. Innovation and change are potentially disruptive and may well be initially viewed in a negative manner, being seen as a threat to the *status quo*, or as creating additional and unnecessary work for staff. The role of communication is therefore vitally important in change management.

9.4   COMMUNICATION DIFFICULTIES ASSOCIATED WITH INNOVATION

All systems resist change and humans are no exception to this rule! Although some staff may readily accept change, others will be less enthusiastic and resistance to organizational change is an almost inevitable reaction among at least some staff. Since innovation is, by definition, fundamental in nature it will necessitate behavioural and attitudinal adjustments by the individuals within an organization. It frequently involves the relinquishment of well-established, familiar and comfortable practices and the adoption of new ones which carry with them feelings of insecurity, vulnerability and perhaps resentment. Some individuals will find the changes difficult to master. Staff perceptions of their role in the change process are very important, since there is a growing body of evidence to indicate that the extent to which an innovation is successfully implemented is in large part determined by individual users' responses to it, and in turn 'users' involvement is manifested chiefly in *communication interactions* related to the innovation' (Lewis and Seibold, 1996, p. 132). Thus, the process of communication becomes central at times of change.

To overcome user resistance, it is essential firstly to identify the exact nature and causes of such resistance. While opposition to innovation is a common phenomenon, it can stem from a variety of reasons, including misunderstanding and lack of knowledge, feelings of fear and inadequacy, or a sense of being threatened. Furthermore, such resistance does not just occur at the outset, but can emerge at any time during the process. Diagnosing the exact nature and source of the resistance or obstacles and taking remedial action can therefore be difficult (see Chapters 3 and 4). Indeed, those opposed to change may keep their dissent covert, since it requires courage for staff overtly to oppose an initiative which is vigorously supported by management.

It is also important to accept that not all resistance is unhelpful. Well founded and constructive criticisms often result in improvements to the innovation or its implementation. Staff should therefore be encouraged to respond honestly and in a spirit of partnership throughout the change process. A necessary first step is that of persuading members that the change will improve current practice. Management need to communicate these advantages clearly throughout the organization and identify problems which create barriers to obtaining accurate employee feedback. Effective two-way channels of communication between the advocates of change and those directly affected by it need to be created to enable any problems to be readily addressed. Deetz (1995, p. 82) has suggested that this approach should be viewed as an attempt to create what he terms 'dialogic communication' within the workplace, and used as a means of expanding participation in the decision-making process. This requires the development of a communication strategy which is educative, facilitative, supportive and participatory.

Involvement in the decision-making process has consistently been recognized as a key strategy for dealing with resistance to change (Kanter, 1983). Staff will be more negatively disposed to an innovation unless they have been actively involved in its formulation, and indeed the concept of power equalization in organizations has been long advocated as a means of countering resistance (Leavitt, 1965). In like vein, Havelock (1969, p. 83) proposed that 'participant involvement may be accepted as a general "Law of Innovation".' The quality of involvement is an important consideration and management need to promote an integrative culture that offers every member of staff the opportunity to contribute meaningfully to the innovation, since difficulties will arise if the process becomes no more than a thin veneer of participation or one of pseudo-consultation.

The evidence suggests that even modest efforts can yield tangible benefits. Aiello (1983), in a survey of top US corporations, found that those which regularly carried out staff attitude surveys had half the rate of industrial stoppages of similar organizations which did not. More recently, Schweiger and Denisi (1991) carried out a controlled study of two worksites facing large scale redundancies. In one of these, the workforce was given extensive information about everything that was happening, while in the other the existing level of information was maintained. Absenteeism and other stress indicators remained significantly lower in the former site throughout the redundancy period. This study indicated that clear information reduces uncertainty, and that high levels of uncertainty reduce the organization's ability to successfully cope with change.

Research by Tourish and Hargie (1996a) and Hargie and Tourish (1996b), examining communicative relationships in the work environment, suggests a positive correlation between the amount of communication people engage in and the development of interpersonal trust. Those within the workplace with whom a greater amount of interaction was carried on received more positive trust evaluations than those with whom contact was less frequent and who were perceived to be more organizationally remote. It has been found that staff place greater trust in communication which they receive from managers if it comes through informal rather than formal communication channels (Johnson et al, 1994), although it has also been noted that managers have a marked propensity to rely on formal methods of approach (Jablin, 1987).

Not surprisingly, at times of organizational change the relationship with immediate managers has been shown to be crucial. Kramer (1995), in a study of staff undergoing significant change in job roles in a range of organizations, found that the relationship between superior and subordinate had a significant impact on the latter's physical, psychological and cognitive adjustment in the new role. The style of management adopted by superiors is therefore of key importance to staff at the operational level.

9.5   OPEN MANAGEMENT AND ORGANIZATIONAL CHANGE

Two contrasting management strategies which are used to maintain and control relationships in organizations can be distinguished (Lee and Jablin, 1995). These are:

(i)   Management by *suppression*. Here the views of subordinates are discouraged, information is viewed as the prerogative of superiors, management perceive their role as directive, communication flows vertically downwards, and decisions are imposed.

(ii) Management by *expression*. By contrast, in this style open discussion is encouraged, information is shared, communication flows in two directions, differences of opinion are regarded as helpful, and the aim is decisions by concurrence.

The latter approach is representative of an open style of management. A fundamental tenet of this style is that organizations are communicative systems whose effectiveness is predicated upon interdependent two-way human relationships. This open style is characterized by both a vertical and lateral communication flow which encourages participative decision making and an open attitude to the flow of information through the promotion of informality. Staff are involved in determining the details of what they do, and in shaping the overall direction of the organization. Managers using an open style will be good listeners, will establish the needs and concerns of staff, will fully explain and clarify actions and decisions, will be supportive and provide verbal and non-verbal rewards. There will also be more use of personal strategies, which are concerned with social rather than task contents, and which include jokes, personal disclosures about life experiences, and the discussion of shared past experiences (Lee and Jablin, 1995).

There is growing evidence to support this management style. For example, one meta-analysis of 43 studies has concluded that profit-sharing, worker ownership and worker participation in decision making are all positively associated with increased productivity (Doucouliagos, 1995).

9.6 INTERNAL COMMUNICATION AND INNOVATIVENESS

The diffusion of innovation within organizations takes place as information is communicated formally and informally (through the 'grapevine'), by individuals and groups. In order for worthwhile progress to be achieved, proposed changes must be effectively communicated and disseminated. This is also influenced by the nature of the organizational culture within which it takes place. Managers have a key role to play in helping to create, promote and transmit the appropriate climate. There are three aspects of organizational climate: (a) oneself, (b) others/colleagues and (c) the organization.

It has been shown that staff who communicate more with their colleagues report less psychological distance between themselves and their organization and express more satisfaction with working relationships (Fink and Chen, 1995). The particular values and decision-making structures which managers espouse and implement can have a key impact on staff perceptions of climate. Innovation and change involve risk. Whether there is a strong fear of failure in the organization or whether risk-taking is encouraged and supported is crucial.

Effective internal communication and receptivity to change are closely linked. Without a culture which encourages open communication, good ideas may not be channelled upwards to those in management who have the responsibility and power to promote and implement them. Poor communication results from bottlenecks and blockages due to inadequate communication systems. A lack of organizational and managerial support creates obstacles which act as major impediments to innovation. Yet there is evidence that many staff within the NHS have given up on attempting to promote suggestions to management, feeling that these get lost within the system and produce no tangible benefits (Tourish and Hargie, 1996b).

Within large organizations such as the NHS, there are often particular problems in innovating which have to be addressed. An increase in size creates a tendency towards greater depersonalization, a more rigid structure and uniform culture. In essence, the difficult dilemma is to encourage an acceptance of change while still sustaining a high degree of organizational integrity. An organic organizational structure, characterized by a flatter hierarchy, more flexible teams and job definitions, and greater opportunities for lateral communication, is more appropriate for facilitating innovation (King and Anderson, 1995).

The successful adoption of an innovation is dependent upon managerial perception of effectiveness, but it is also important that management expectations are successfully communicated to those whose acceptance and cooperation are necessary for making the innovation work (Damanpour, 1990). This creates a mutual expectancy of high performance, since the positive impact which credible high expectations have on performance, when they are communicated by figures of authority who genuinely believe in them, has been widely noted in the literature (e.g. Eden, 1993). When asked to identify the most frequent problems which they encounter, managers tend to focus on matters relating to interpersonal relationships (Hargie et al, 1994b). For managers to act as effective change agents, it is therefore necessary that they have at their disposal appropriate communicative skills and strategies.

Poor interpersonal relationships and low job satisfaction are incompatible with the creation of a culture of total quality management. What, therefore, must be done? To begin with, there is a need for hard data on existing communication relationships before sweeping new initiatives are proposed. The most important reason for this is that managers cannot rely on their own perceptions to give them a comprehensive, objective and accurate picture of communicative behaviours, since they often overrate the effectiveness of their communication practices, and that of their organizations. There is nothing surprising or reprehensible in this. Psychologists have established that through a process termed cognitive dissonance we all tend to search for positive feedback on decisions made and are more likely not to hear negative feedback. Another factor is that groupthink can occur, in that managers are often told what subordinates think they want to hear – a process which has been termed the boss's illusion (Baumeister, 1989). One method of dispensing with such illusions is through the use of communication audits which provide 'an objective picture of what is happening compared with what senior executives think (or have been told) is happening' (Hurst, 1991, p. 24). Such knowledge empowers managers to realistically appraise how communication relationships can best be transformed to meet the needs of the organization.

9.7 AUDITING ORGANIZATIONAL COMMUNICATION

The proposal that organizations should gather data about actual communication practices is still relatively novel in the UK. However, organizations in the US have a richer tradition of developing techniques for assessing how effectively managers and staff interact with each other (e.g. Goldhaber and Rogers, 1979; Downs, 1988).

As this book illustrates, the term audit is now widely used within the NHS. This concept has been extended to the communication function. It is therefore useful to examine how communication audits compare to other audits already operative in the health service. Financial audits are long established, and in recent years terms such as medical audit, clinical audit and organization audit have filtered into the vocabulary of the organization. These have the following common characteristics:

1. *The accumulation of information.* In the case of finance, the goal is to check the efficacy of financial accounting procedures by sampling a representative cross section of transactions within the organization. This might be termed the diagnostic phase of the auditing process.
2. *The creation of management systems.* Systems are developed to control the flow of information and resources over a given period. The auditing of practice in the surgical sphere, for example, focuses on areas such as existing activity rates, theatre capacity and future potential. Systems can then be developed to maximize throughput and take up rates. This is the prescriptive phase of the audit process.
3. *Accountability.* A finance audit ensures that funds are appropriately managed and that efficient methods of financial management are being applied.

Organizations require all three of these strands to be applied to their internal and external communication systems. Given the propensity of communication systems to breakdown, at untold organizational cost, a strong case can be made for taking whatever steps are required to ascertain their general level of effectiveness. Managers need to know who they are communicating with, through what channels and with what productive and qualitative effect. Proper systems must be developed to achieve these goals. Lastly, there should be some accountability for the flow of information within the organization. At a practical level, this means that if vital information is not getting through to its key target audiences, the blockages in the channels of communication must be identified and dealt with.

Accordingly, a communication audit can be defined as: 'a comprehensive and thorough study of communication philosophy, concepts, structure, flow and practice within an organisation' (Emmanuel, 1985, p. 50). It tells organizations:

- Who you *should* communicate with.
- Who you *actually do* communicate with.
- What you *should* be communicating.
- How you *should* communicate with them.
- How you *actually do* communicate with them.

(Bland and Jackson, 1990, p. 142)

Comparisons between communication and other audits raise a number of important methodological issues. On the surface, communication audits would appear to deal with less tangible issues than, for example, those dealt with by a finance audit team. However, Amernic (1992, p. 4) points out that even within such apparently solid areas as financial accounting 'Management has considerable discretion within generally accepted accounting principles, and indeed may implement a chosen principle in a variety of ways'. This means that documents such as a company's annual reports are in effect an interpretation of selected data. Given the enormous amount of financial transactions which occur, there is really little alternative to this. Like all such exercises, the data may be skewed (intentionally or otherwise) by the prejudices or imperatives of the individuals involved in its selection. Systems guard against this, but do so within limits.

When one considers the vast array of communicative contacts in even small businesses, any effort to chart all of these would be almost impossible. To do so would necessitate analysing every single face-to-face or telephone conversation, and examining every written memorandum, fax and letter. Such an approach would cost a prohibitive amount, overwhelm researchers with data, pose ethical dilemmas and interfere with the day-to-day functioning of the organization. It should be pointed out, however, that for a very small, self-contained, section of an organization, a full and comprehensive audit is possible. For example, Skipper (1992) carried out an audit of a dysphasia clinic within a large hospital, in which she analysed written communications with patients, video-recorded the clinic sessions and interviewed all the staff, patients and relatives who attended the clinic over a set period of time. The results of this audit provided valuable data for the subsequent evaluation of the quality of this particular service provision. In most instances, however, it is necessary to develop a sampling frame which will provide organizations with a selected, yet valid and reliable, account of their communication practices. This necessitates selecting a representative, stratified, sample of the workforce (i.e. a sample population genuinely representative of the key groups within the organization) as the basis for data collection.

9.8   COMMUNICATION AUDIT MEASURES

The measures employed in any particular audit will vary depending upon the exact measurement objectives. In general terms, however, audit measures available include: questionnaires administered to participants asking them to evaluate current communication practices and to identify areas of strengths and weaknesses and suggest how improvements could be effected (similar information can, of course, be obtained from interviews or focus groups); audio or video recordings of interpersonal encounters followed by analysis and evalua-

tion of these recordings; live observation of such episodes *in situ*; 'agent pro-
vocateur' visits; diary analysis to ascertain whom individuals have interacted
with and how often over a given period of time; and self-recordings on paper
by participants following each of their communicative activities. It is useful to
examine each of these methods briefly and to highlight their relative advantages and disadvantages.

9.8.1 Questionnaires

There are existing validated questionnaires which can be readily adapted for
use in any specific communication audit context (Goldhaber and Rogers, 1979;
Downs, 1988). Such questionnaires should form an important part of most
audits, especially in large organizations where the sample population is numer-
ous and it would be impossible to interview everyone. Questionnaires enable
the auditor to obtain the views of a large sample of respondents. They also
allow for a high degree of control over the focus of the research; provide
quantitative data which act as benchmarks against which future performance
can be measured; and the scores can be converted into approval ratings for each
element of the organization under scrutiny (Hargie and Tourish, 1996c). At the
same time, the use of one or more open questions can provide freedom of
expression for respondents to air their wider views (Tourish and Hargie,
1996b).

Audit questionnaires cover attitudes to the volume, timeliness and quality of
communications sent to and received from various sources through different
channels. However, they should also reflect organization-specific communication issues. This will necessitate conducting in-depth interviews with staff from
the different sections of the organization in order to ascertain core themes for
analysis. The objective should be to discover the key issues which people at
various levels within the organization feel they should be communicating about
for inclusion in the questionnaire.

While a well-designed questionnaire is a user-friendly research instrument, it is
not without data collection problems. For example, there is often a low
response rate to postal questionnaires. One method of improving response is
for the organization to sanction the completion of questionnaires in paid working time, at a venue under the auditors' supervision. This signifies a high level
of commitment by the organization to the exercise (itself a valuable gain),
means that the questionnaire is less likely to be seen as another imposition
on top of a busy work schedule and results in as close to a 100% response
rate as it is possible to achieve. The cost to the organization is no more than
1 hour of each person's time (Hargie and Tourish, 1993).

9.8.2   Interviews

The structured interview is a tried and tested approach to data collection (Millar et al, 1992), but it is also time-consuming, and therefore costly. In most instances, it is not feasible to interview every person in the sample. What can be done is to select, usually on the basis of questionnaire responses, a small representative sub-sample and conduct follow-up interviews to obtain more in-depth views about particular issues. Another drawback of interviews as opposed to questionnaires is that the responses obtained are obviously not anonymous, and they can therefore be more restrictive. However, given a trusting relationship between interviewer and interviewee coupled with firm guarantees of confidentiality, they are a valuable data collection tool.

9.8.3   Focus groups

These are, in some respects, an extension of interviews, and have been defined as 'a discussion based interview that produces a particular type of qualitative data' (Millward, 1995, p. 275). Normally, between five and eight individuals of representative staff are selected for participation in small group discussion. The general focus of the discussion is led by a facilitator, although the emphasis is upon allowing members as much freedom as possible to verbalize their thoughts and feelings. The discussion is recorded either on tape or by a collea-gue of the facilitator, and later content analysed for recurring themes. Focus groups are widely used in many forms of communications research (Lunt and Livingstone, 1996). Their chief advantages are that they provide individuals with the opportunity to spark ideas off one another, to try to reach a consensus on identified core issues, and to produce creative solutions to identified pro-blems.

9.8.4   Recordings of interpersonal encounters

One of the most objective methods for obtaining information about commu-nication practices is to record interactive episodes on audio- or video-tape. This then provides an accurate record of what actually occurred during face-to-face encounters. One disadvantage of this approach is that it can be intrusive, and indeed the awareness of being recorded may actually alter the behaviour of those being recorded. Where the recordings involve members of the public there is the added difficulty of obtaining permission to tape their conversations. Despite these drawbacks, recordings have been carried out in a number of different contexts, including doctor's surgeries (Byrne and Long, 1976), com-munity pharmacies (Hargie et al, 1993), speech therapy clinics (Saunders and

Caves, 1986) and hospital wards (MacLeod Clark, 1982). These recordings facilitate an accurate analysis of the behaviours of those involved.

9.8.5 Diary analysis

A simple and readily available method for obtaining information concerning communication contacts is to ask members of staff to analyse their diary entries over a set period of time (Breakwell and Wood, 1995). This will provide an overview of whom they have interacted with, how often, about what topics and for what duration. The problem here is that usually it is only formal meetings and contacts which are entered into diaries, and so other information will not be included.

9.8.6 Self-reports of interactive episodes

A final method for gathering audit information is to employ some form of proforma or schedule on which participants itemize details of all of their communicative activities over a set period (Hargie and Tourish, 1996b). An entry is made by the respondent as soon as possible after each communicative episode. Respondents are asked to list the source of the communication, the topic, the channel (whether telephone, face-to-face, letter, memo, fax etc.), the length of the communication (in pages) or the duration (in minutes), whether it was one- or two-way, and finally to rate the effectiveness of the communication using a scale from one (totally ineffective) to seven (totally effective).

These, then, are the main methods which can be used to audit organizational communication. Decisions about which methods to employ will depend upon a range of factors, including the purpose and scale of the audit, the accessibility of respondents and their responsiveness to being recorded.

9.9   COMMUNICATION AUDIT OUTCOMES

Hargie et al (1994c) have reviewed the results of a number of NHS audits. From these it is possible to garner several recurring themes about communication.

9.9.1   Lack of information

It is clear that employees desire, and appreciate, being fully informed about key issues affecting their organization, and in particular those which will have a direct bearing upon their jobs. While there was a great deal of goodwill and commitment expressed by staff, one of the consistent complaints was that of people feeling underinformed, and, by implication, undervalued. Given the well-known adage that information is power, lack of information understandably results in a feeling of disempowerment. The *pace of change* was another issue which concerned staff, and as discussed earlier, during such change periods it is even more vital that staff feel fully (and honestly) informed about what is happening or is about to happen. While the pace of NHS change is often externally driven and outside the control of management, its impact can be lessened by ensuring that staff are informed as soon as possible about what changes will occur, when, and what the implications are likely to be.

9.9.2   Power of the grapevine

Where information is not forthcoming from management, staff will invent it! In all organizations, there are creative individuals who, building upon minimal information, construct plausible scenarios about decisions which are supposed to have already been made. In the absence of definite data to the contrary, it is not surprising that credence is given to this alternative source from the grapevine. A recurrent finding was strong reliance on the grapevine on the part of staff, and correspondingly less reliance on information from management. The grapevine will flourish in organizations where staff are selectively informed on a 'need to know' basis. To circumvent worst-case stories contaminating the organization, firm communication channels must be established for the dissemination of information.

9.9.3   Timeliness of information

There was a view amongst staff that information was not being delivered early enough, and this was especially the case in those organizations spanning several different geographical locations. Mechanisms must therefore be established to ensure a swift flow of information. Organizations should develop free-flowing 'communication highways' along which messages can be delivered both speedily and accurately, and without encountering bottlenecks or roadblocks. Furthermore, all staff should have ready access to this highway. One way of achieving this is to appoint communication drivers (or communication champions) who will deliver the information within their own area. This means that organizations need to identify and train enthusiastic individuals who will be trusted and respected by their peers, and use these individuals to both gather information from their colleagues about attitudes to communication and to deliver relevant information to them. These drivers, in turn, should form part of an overall communications team which would meet on a regular basis and have an input into executive decision-making. With these approaches, it might be more possible to avoid the multiple pile-ups which seem to bedevil so much organizational communication at present.

9.9.4 Upwards communication

A major survey has shown that while chief executives in trusts and health authorities recognized the importance of good upward communication, in practice 25% of trusts and 20% of health authorities who responded did not cite this as one of their objectives for internal communication strategies (Lloyd, 1994). Yet the findings from Hargie et al (1994c) illustrate the importance which staff attach to upwards communication. In particular, staff were keen to report on initiatives taken in their area and wanted to be able to request any information they felt was necessary for them to do their job effectively. They also felt that more action should be taken on information which they were providing, with the greatest need for follow-up felt to be from senior managers. In other words, lip service should not be paid to this area, since if no follow-up occurs, cynicism soon sets in. Another issue which was raised was the need for a climate in which bottom-up communication was fostered and seen as positive, since there was a fear that if someone spoke the truth, in terms of giving critical views, they might then be marked by senior managers.

9.9.5 Channels of communication

In some instances, it was clear that there was a heavy reliance upon written communication, whereas a strong preference emerged for face-to-face communication wherever possible. Newsletters were not highly valued, since they often contained large amounts of what was seen as irrelevant or cosmetic information and were also perceived to be a costly exercise. However, shorter and more specialized bulletin sheets or factsheets were more favourably received. Notice boards were rarely examined, since they were seen as being overposted, disorganized and covered with out-of-date or useless notices. To avoid this chaos, if a notice board is deemed to be important, someone should be given responsibility for its management. Another common complaint was that boards were often seen to be in the wrong location. Humans, like all animals, are territorial – we do not like to stray too far away from our habitual lairs and paths. Managers need to take cognizance of this and bring the boards to the staff rather than expecting the reverse to happen.

9.9.6   Location versus organization

Where an organization spanned several sites, the first loyalty tended to be to the geographic location rather that the corporate identity. This was especially marked where the sites were formerly independent entities. Managers need to appreciate the importance of place in such situations. It is positive that staff have a bond to their workplace which they are reluctant to relinquish, since it would not be desirable to have staff with no real depth of commitment to their organization. A sense of corporate identity can be fostered by developing cross-site teams where possible. Also, as new staff are appointed, with no prior allegiance-baggage, the staff induction programme should ensure that corporate loyalty is fostered.

9.9.7   Visibility of senior managers

Senior managers often engage in activities to encourage communication with staff on the shop floor – for example, management by walking about. However, there are several possible drawbacks to this approach. When prior notice is given, it can be given red carpet treatment when all of the benches are scrubbed and the floors well polished as the senior manager inspects the area – in essence this becomes management by walking past! Conversely, when the senior person arrives unannounced, there is evidence that such informal contacts are often viewed with suspicion by staff, who may interpret this as a form of snooping or assessment. At the same time, our audits have revealed that staff do want to receive talks from, and interface with, senior managers. Three of the comments from staff on one of the audits were: 'We would like to know what senior managers look like'; 'The bosses are just names' and 'Senior managers should appear at team briefs occasionally to hear staff's point of view'. It seems that the solution here is for senior managers to arrange formal face-to-face meetings with groups of staff, at least once a year but preferably biannually, at which there is an opportunity for any issue to be raised. There should be a formal informality about these contacts – they should be round table, over coffee, for a set period (no more than 1 hour), should begin with a statement from the senior manager, and open out to allow anyone to raise any topic. This not only allows senior executives to 'address the troops', but also helps to foster a sense of openness and accessibility within the organization. There would seem to be a cathartic effect in being listened to by those in positions of power and this should be facilitated by organizations. In other words, communication at these meetings should very definitely be two-way.

9.9.8 Unproductive meetings

There was a feeling, especially among middle managers, that there were too many unnecessary meetings, at which little of importance was decided. The disease of meetingitis has taken hold in many organizations. A good analogy here is between this type of meeting and a rain dance: an elaborate ritual is performed and the central characters may enjoy the performance, but the activity has no direct impact upon the outcome for which it is intended. Meetings should therefore be carefully monitored – a strict guillotine should operate so that they do not drag on interminably, and groups should be given a few specific and measurable goals to achieve in the meeting.

9.9.9 Communication skills training

There was a strong view expressed that senior managers throughout the organization should undertake communication skills training (CST). This form of training, which has been shown to be effective across a range of professional contexts (Hargie, 1997), should be organization specific and should focus on how interactions with staff can be conducted in the most supportive and encouraging manner. In particular, existing management development programmes should be reviewed in order to sharpen their focus on CST so that all managers can gain exposure to a common skills base in this important area of their work.

9.9.10 Annual communications review

A procedure should be implemented to allow the organization to review existing practices, processes and patterns of communication. This would involve representatives from all locations attending a 1- or 2-day workshop, and would encompass 'bottom up' as well as 'top down' appraisal. The recommendations from the communications review would then represent a focused communication strategy for the organization.

9.10 DEVELOPING A COMMUNICATION STRATEGY

A communication strategy is a process which enables managers to evaluate the communication consequences of the decision-making process, and which integrates this into the normal business planning cycle and psyche of the organization (Tourish and Hargie, 1996c). There are four key stages in the development of such a strategy.

1. *Secure senior management commitment.* This is the cornerstone of change in any organization. A starting point is for management to devise its own programme of standards on communication, and then share this with the wider organization. What do the standards mean in practice? How will every organizational unit be transformed if they are implemented? What has stopped such implementation in the past? How much can be agreed and how much will remain in dispute for the foreseeable future? What training needs arise? How quickly can change begin?
2. *Identify current practice.* Managers need to start from a clear picture of where the organization is in communication terms. This means that some form of audit of existing communication practices must be carried out before any attempt to formulate a strategy.
3. *Set standards to measure success.* This operates on two levels. It should be clear that the organization is not concerned only with improving communication for its own sake. This means habituating managers and staff to the following questions: what are the key business problems that reflect our communication difficulties? What are our major communication problems? What changes are required to eliminate these problems? What targets can we set to eliminate the problems that arise from communication failure? What targets can be set to eliminate communication failure itself?

   In addition, staff satisfaction with communication is important for its own sake. If existing communication practice has been thoroughly evaluated, then targets can also be set for:

   • Increased and sustained knowledge.
   • High levels of goodwill and credibility.
   • A regular flow of communication.
   • Accurate expectations about future milestones in organizational development (i.e. fewer toxic shocks).
   • Satisfaction with levels of participation.

   Ongoing audit research will track the progress of all these factors.
4. *Incorporate this process* into the business planning cycle (and psyche) of the organization. A genuine communication strategy means involving all managers and ultimately all staff in identifying goals, standards of good practice and methods of evaluation. The starting point is the requirement that when business plans are being drawn up, the communication consequences of plans are considered. Therefore, it is suggested that at the business planning stage managers and staff routinely address, in a very non-routine way, the following issues:

   • What are the communication or information implications of the decision-making process? Again, this should not be only a top down process. It is quite feasible to consult staff at all levels on this issue. The threats and opportunities which this poses should also be considered.

- What will people need to know about the implications of this policy decision? This could encompass people internal and external to the organization.
- Who is going to be responsible for spreading the information (i.e. what source of communication will be appropriate)? Communication is primarily a management responsibility, but need not involve only managers. Empowerment here must mean involving staff in the setting of standards and procedures for communication.
- How will this information be communicated – face to face, through written memorandum, through group meetings (i.e. what channels of communication will be used)?
- What is the absolute essence of the information that will be required (i.e. what is the nature of the message that we will be spreading)?
- What mechanisms exist to consult and involve people? How can they be strengthened? Has team briefing degenerated into an empty ritual or is it still effective? Does it contain any facility for staff to feed information back up the management line?
- How can we promote greater informality within the organization? Specifically, how many bureaucratic procedures can we eliminate?
- What personal behavioural changes can managers make right away to facilitate a new pro-communications culture? How should managers be facilitated to honestly identify their own strengths and weaknesses as communicators, motivators and, ultimately, leaders?
- Within this framework, and assuming top management involvement, a basis can be laid for transforming patterns of communication, organizational structures, levels of involvement and, ultimately, key business outcomes.

9.11 CONCLUSION

Effective communication is both a key determinant of organizational success and a crucial factor in any attempt at organizational innovation. Change is essentially a social process requiring the active participation and willing cooperation of those affected. Consequently, in order to maximize the chances of successful implementation, it is necessary to develop effective systems of internal communications that will promote members' acceptance and involvement. An important dimension of this is a managerial style which fosters openness and honesty across all levels of the organization. A well developed, clearly formulated communication strategy is a vital ingredient of effective change management. Part of such a strategy should be a regular audit of internal communications.

9.12 SUMMARY POINTS

- At times of change and innovation communication needs increase.
- The NHS has gone through a period of enormous change.
- Research in the NHS has shown varying levels of staff dissatisfaction with existing communications.
- Improved internal communications lead to a range of positive outcomes for the organization.
- Satisfaction with communication improves with empowerment and involvement.
- Communication audits allow managers to identify best practice and to diagnose existing problems.
- There are many practical tools for collecting data in communication audits.
- Staff should be involved in the audit process.
- The audit should form part of an overall communications strategy.

ACKNOWLEDGEMENT

Many of the ideas contained in this chapter were generated by our late colleague, friend and brother, Colin Thomas Cecil Hargie, 1948–1996, and we therefore dedicate this chapter to him.

REFERENCES

Aiello R (1983) Employee attitude surveys: impact on corporate decisions. *Public Relations Journal* **7**:21.

Albrow M (1992) Sine Ira et Studio – or do organisations have feelings? *Organization Studies* **13**:313–329.

Amernic J (1992) A case study of corporate financial accounting: Massey-Ferguson's visible accounting decisions. *Critical Perspectives on Accounting* **3**:1–43.

Barker J and Tompkins P (1994) Identification in the self-managing organization: Characteristics of target and tenure. *Human Communication Research* **21**:223–240.

Baumeister R (1989) Motives and costs of self-presentation in organizations. In: Giacalone RA and Rosenfeld P (editors) *Impression Management in the Organization*. Hillsdale, NJ: Erlbaum.

Bland M and Jackson P (1990) *Effective Employee Communications*. London: Kogan Page.

Breakwell G and Wood P (1995) Diary techniques. In: Breakwell G, Hammond S and Fife-Schaw C (editors) *Research Methods in Psychology*. London: Sage.

Byrne P and Long B (1976) *Doctors Talking To Patients*. London: HMSO.

Church AH (1994) The character of organizational communication: a review and new conceptualization. *The International Journal of Organizational Analysis* **2**:18–53.

Clampitt P and Downs C (1993) Employee perceptions of the relationship between communication and productivity: a field study. *Journal of Business Communication* **30**:5–28.

Damanpour F (1990) Innovation effectiveness, adoption and organizational performance. In: West MA and Farr JL (editors) *Innovation and Creativity at Work*. Chichester: Wiley.

Deetz S (1995) *Transforming Communication, Transforming Business: Building Responsive and Responsible Workplaces*. New Jersey: Hampton Press.

Dickson D, Hargie O and Morrow N (1997) *Communication Skills Training for Health Professionals*. Second edition. London: Chapman and Hall.

Doucouliagos C (1995) Worker participation and productivity in labor-managed and participatory capitalist forms: a meta-analysis. *Industrial and Labor Relations Review* **49**:58–77.

Downs C (1988) *Communication Audits*. London: Harper Collins.

Drucker PF (1985) *Innovation and Entrepreneurship: Practice and Principles*. London: Heinemann.

Eden D (1993) Interpersonal expectations in organizations. In: Blanck P (editor) *Interpersonal Expectations: Theory, Research and Applications*. Cambridge: Cambridge University Press.

Emmanuel M (1985) Auditing communication practices. In: Reuss C and Silvas D (editors) *Inside Organizational Communication*. Second edition. New York: Longman.

Fink EL and Chen S (1995) A Galileo analysis of organizational climate. *Human Communication Research* **21**:494–521.

Goldhaber G and Rogers D (1979) *Auditing Organizational Communication Systems*. Texas: Kendall-Hunt.

Grint K (1994) Reengineering history: social resonances and business process reengineering. *Organization* **1**:179–201.

Hanson G (1986) *Determinants of Firm Performance: an Integration of Economic and Organizational Factors*. Unpublished doctoral dissertation, University of Michigan Business School.

Hargie O (1997) Training in communication skills: research, theory and practice. In: Hargie O (editor) *The Handbook of Communication Skills*. Second edition. London: Routledge.

Hargie O and Tourish D (1993) Assessing the effectiveness of communication in organisations: the communication audit approach. *Health Services Management Research* **6**:276–285.

Hargie C and Tourish D (1996a) Corporate communication in the management of innovation and change. *Corporate Communications: An International Journal* **1**:3–11.

Hargie O and Tourish D (1996b) Auditing communication practices to improve the management of human resources: an inter-organisational study. *Health Services Management Research* **9**:209–222.

Hargie O and Tourish D (1996c) Auditing internal communication to build business success. *Internal Communication Focus* November 1996, 10–14.

Hargie O, Morrow N and Woodman C (1993) *Looking Into Community Pharmacy: Identifying Effective Communication Skills in Pharmacist–Patient Consultations*. Jordanstown: University of Ulster

Hargie O, Saunders C and Dickson D (1994a) *Social Skills in Interpersonal Communication*. Third edition. London: Routledge.

Hargie C, Tourish D and Hargie O (1994b) Managers communicating: an investigation of core situations and difficulties within educational organizations. *The International Journal of Educational Management* **8**:23–28.

Hargie O, Tourish D, Waldrop-White C and Marshall B (1994c) Did you hear it on the grapevine? *Health Service Journal* **104**:26–29.

Havelock RG (editor) (1969) *Planning for Innovation Through Dissemination and Utilization of Knowledge*. Ann Arbor, Michigan: Center for Research on Utilization of Scientific Knowledge.

Hurst B (1991) *The Handbook of Communication Skills*. London: Kogan Page.

Jablin F (1987) Formal organization structure. In: Jablin F, Putnam L, Roberts K and Porter L (editors) *Handbook of Organizational Communication*. Newbury Park: Sage.

Johnson J, Donohue W, Atkin C and Johnson S (1994) Differences between formal and informal communication channels. *Journal of Business Communication* **31**:111–122.

Kanter RM (1983) *The Change Masters*. New York: Free Press.

King N and Anderson N (1995) *Innovation and Change in Organizations*. London: Routledge.

Kramer MW (1995) A longitudinal study of superior-subordinate communication during job transfers. *Human Communication Research* **22**:39–64.

Leavitt HJ (1965) Applied organizational change in industry: structural, technological and humanistic approaches. In: March JA (editor) *Handbook of Organizations*. Chicago: Rand McNally.

Lee J and Jablin F (1995) Maintenance communication in superior-subordinate work relationships. *Human Communication Research* **22**:220–257.

Lewis LK and Seibold DR (1996) Communication during intraorganizational innovation adoption: predicting users' behavioral coping responses to innovations in organizations. *Communication Monographs* **63**:131–157.

Lloyd P (1994) Hard news. *Health Service Journal* **104**:19.

Lunt P and Livingstone S (1996) Rethinking the focus group in media and communications research. *Journal of Communication* **46**:79–98.

MacLeod Clark J (1982) *Nurse–Patient Verbal Interaction: An Analysis of Recorded Conversations from Selected Surgical Wards*. PhD Thesis, University of London.

Millar R, Crute V and Hargie O (1992) *Professional Interviewing*. London: Routledge.

Millward L (1995) Focus groups. In: Breakwell G, Hammond S and Fife-Schaw C (editors) *Research Methods in Psychology*. London: Sage.

Saunders C and Caves R (1986) An empirical approach to the identification of communication skills with reference to speech therapy. *Journal of Further and Higher Education* **10**:29–44.

Schweiger D and Denisi A (1991) Communicating with employees: a longitudinal field experiment. *Academy of Management Journal* **34**:110–135.

Skipper M (1992) *Communication Processes and their Effectiveness in the Management and Treatment of Dysphagia*. DPhil Thesis, University of Ulster, Jordanstown.

Slappendel, C. (1996) Perspectives on innovation in organizations. *Organization Studies* **17**:107–129.

Smith A (1991) *Innovative Employee Communication: New Approaches to Improving Trust, Teamwork and Performance*. Englewood Cliffs: Prentice-Hall.

Tourish D and Hargie O (1993) Quality assurance and internal organizational communications. *International Journal of Health Care Quality Assurance* **6**:22–28.

Tourish D and Hargie O (1996a) Communication audits and the management of change: a case study from an NHS trust. *Health Services Management Research* **9**:125–135.

Tourish D and Hargie O (1996b) Communication in the NHS: using qualitative approaches to analyse effectiveness. *Journal of Management in Medicine* **10**:38–54.

Tourish D and Hargie C (1996c) Internal communication: key steps in evaluating and improving performance. *Corporate Communications* **1**:11–16.

Walker J and Henry D (1991) *Managing Innovation*. London: Sage.

West MA and Farr JA (editors) (1990) *Innovation and Creativity at Work*. Chichester: Wiley.

Chapter 10

GETTING THE MESSAGE ACROSS – LANGUAGE, TRANSLATION, MARKETING AND SELLING

Rosalind Eve and Paul Hodgkin

10.1 INTRODUCTION

Since 1994, the Framework for Appropriate Care Throughout Sheffield (FACTS) project team have been working, with some success, to implement evidence-based change on a city-wide scale.

Getting people to change what they have always done is not easy. Usually, it cannot be commanded from above, and if it is, then all too often the results are unpredictable and at worst, counter-productive. Nor are most people, including those for whom this book is written, in a position to offer incentives, induce-ments, money, expense account lunches or any of the other magical trinkets which sometimes ease the wheels of commerce. The experience of the FACTS project team has taught us that the first step to bringing about any change successfully depends, first and foremost, on the change agent's ability to com-prehend and appreciate the myriad factors that effect change, and their ability to address the obstacles to change and to work within the shifting sands of real world, chaotic, unpredictable complexity.

This chapter sets out some of the lessons learnt by the FACTS team. We begin by exploring the language commonly used in the health service, trying to identify the gaps in thinking about how best to bring about change in clinical behaviour. We then go on to consider how marketing techniques might help to bridge some of those gaps.

Implementing Change With Clinical Audit. Edited by Richard Baker, Hilary Hearnshaw and Noelle Robertson.
© 1999 John Wiley & Sons, Ltd.

10.2   THE LANGUAGE OF DEVELOPMENT

Language infects and inflects our thought at every level (Dennett, 1993)

Language shapes how we think. In particular, metaphors are ubiquitous in language, and universally structure what and how we think (Lakoff and Johnson, 1980). For example the underlying metaphor 'up is good/down is bad' grounds all of the following:

He felt low, she was on top of the world, high flyer, weighed down with sadness, things are looking up, laid low.

Such examples may seem trivial. The insidious way in which metaphors structure thought, however, becomes clear with the language that we use to describe emotions:

Floods of tears, all steamed up, boiling over with anger, exploding with rage, emotionally incontinent, frigid, ventilating feelings, the flow of emotions.

Here the language is structured around the metaphor 'emotions are dangerous fluids'. This metaphor is never explicit. Yet if you think about the language we use when talking about emotions, it is clearly structured around the notion of emotions as dangerous fluids. And this metaphor makes some lines of thought – for example, the need to control and contain emotions – much more natural and congenial than others. Professionals in particular are often explicitly taught to maintain distance and not to become over-involved. Whilst such an approach clearly has some merit, it tends to shut off other ways of viewing feelings. For example, the basic dynamic involved in emotional interactions could usefully be structured around the metaphor of resonance: if you feel sad or angry, it is likely that sooner or later I will begin to feel sad or angry, too. Emotions then become data which enrich understanding of the other, rather than something to be feared.

Nor are scientific and rational concepts exempt from the insights and limitations of the language in which it is expressed. Within medicine the commonest metaphor is 'medicine is war' (Hodgkin, 1985):

The body's defences, overwhelming infection, heart attack, casualty, House Officer, therapeutic armamentarium, LD-50, cohort, infiltrating disease, killer T cells, the war on cancer, aggressive therapy, he's lost the battle.

Medicine would be very different if it took 'medicine is collaboration' or 'healing is balance' as its main structuring metaphor.

Research and development too have their metaphors and as with everything, make some ways of thinking about R&D more likely than others. This section explores the way we limit our thinking about changing behaviour in the health service.

10.2.1 Research

Re-searching literally means going over again that which is known in order to discover the underlying 'truth'. The idealized activity is that of drawing away Nature's veil by means of a singular defining experiment. Much of the language of research is modelled around court room dramas: trials are conducted, cases studied, findings contested, evidence weighed, lines of inquiry followed, and judgement suspended until the hard facts are in or the incontestable truth is established. And Justice herself sees blindness as desirable just as investigators do. Interestingly, the idealized output of the legal process – justice – is seen to be an entirely worthy end in and of itself. The legal profession is careful to distance itself from any consequences – such as punishment – which may flow from its deliberations. Similarly, the research process has an idealized output – truth – which requires no further action or justification.

For researchers the payoff, in this metaphor, is some variant of the Nobel prize, i.e. public acknowledgement by peers that one has identified a truth that no one else has yet identified, and that one's contribution to the sum of knowledge has indeed been original. Whilst the metaphor may have utility, it also constrains how we think. Researchers 'searching for the truth' see implementation as a very secondary issue, and the task of development itself comes to be seen as searching for those techniques of implementation which will hold true for all circumstances.

10.2.2 Development

Development is usually thought of as consisting of those processes which take research through into some useful tool (Black and Mays, 1996). Historically, this notion took root after the Second World War, when basic science was systematically and rapidly transformed into weapons such as radar. Development, in this metaphor, is essentially using engineering to work out how to apply 'basic' or pure knowledge. A working, commercially viable product, ready to hand on to the sales and marketing team is the *end* of the process. How such a product is actually used is of little concern to the R&D department.

10.2.3 Dissemination

Dissemination is derived from the notion of 'sowing seeds'. Scatter as many papers/newspaper articles etc. as possible, most will fail, or fall on infertile ground, but some will take root. Like pearls before swine, this metaphor places responsibility for acting on the truth on to the shoulders of those lucky enough to have the Gospel showered on them from above. It assumes that the main impediment to rational people implementing the evidence is that they have not heard the truth. With the more enlightened dissemination methods adopted by, for example, the Centre for Reviews and Dissemination, there has been a welcome trend towards making the evidence more accessible to busy clinicians. All too often, however, hints of older attitudes remain: the pearls may have been nicely polished but assumptions about clinicians and why they don't 'act on the evidence' remain unchanged.

10.2.4   Implementation

The underlying metaphor here is that there should be an 'implement' (sharp or blunt) which can be used to change the process of medical care, or maybe, to hit the relevant professionals over the head. In the past implementation has relied on common sense – the rational adoption of rational information because it makes sense, or, if that didn't work, try directives. Finally, if all else failed, financial incentives have been resorted to – but they are expensive and may produce unpredictable results (Morone, 1986). In recent years, more sophisticated implements have been developed, such as total quality management, guidelines and audit. At their best, each of these methods is successful in bringing about improvement and developing a culture of change. However, as with the standard R&D metaphor, there is danger in relying on the application of one 'true' method of implementation, whichever that may be.

10.2.5   The poorly (performing) doctor

Doctors who fail to do 'the right thing' are seen metaphorically as sick. Medicine is a rational endeavour, so the argument goes, practised by rational clinicians. Change is simply a matter of getting the facts through to them. Failure to act rationally must be a sign of sickness. The standard response to sickness is to prescribe some therapy, and so guidelines or some other intervention are administered to the poorly docs in the hope that they will mend their ways and return to the norm(al).

10.2.6   Marketing

The essential metaphor of the market is of free agents engaging in trade: bustle and barrow boys, share traders, excitement, the adjustment of the truth for commercial gain and *caveat emptor*. Marketing brings a more pro-active shape to the idea of bringing about change – go out and sell, create markets, manipulate them and the customers. Mixed in are militaristic and sexual metaphors: battling for market share, market penetration, sales force, being the dominant force in the market place, the cut and thrust of competition, having a sexy product, etc.

Marketing itself is still clearly focused on a product – within its commercial definition it is about satisfying customer needs with a flow of products. Herein lie many of the limitations of its uses within the NHS. Most changes in health care require complex, simultaneous adjustments by most players. Marketing can be used either to promote the change as a whole or to sell particular facets of the change.

Whilst it has achieved considerable success in changing prescribing behaviour in the past, marketing will only work in conjunction with a whole range of other work (Grol, 1997). Nonetheless, marketing, as we all know from our daily lives, does have tremendous power. This power derives from firstly analysing the context in which change will take place, and secondly working with the motivations of those who will enact the change. Success depends upon getting these two factors right.

10.3   USING MARKETING AND SELLING TECHNIQUES

Changing clinical behaviour, by adapting the marketing techniques used by the pharmaceutical industry, is well established in the US (Soumerai and Avorn, 1990; see Chapter 1), and marketing principles are increasingly gaining credibility in this country (Dawson, 1995; Dickinson, 1995). Marketing is industry's method of implementation: in a commercial context it is self-evident that once a product has been successfully developed, it needs marketing and selling.

Whilst marketing may have acquired some acceptability over the last 5 years, selling still remains a largely alien concept. How can selling with all its brash pushiness possibly help clinicians in their dispassionate assessment of what constitutes the right course of action?

The FACTS team have adapted both marketing and selling to promote change. By comparison with methods currently being used by the pharmaceutical industry, the techniques we have used are somewhat unsophisticated (and a great deal cheaper). Nonetheless, we believe our experience has some valuable messages for others embarking on similar work.

10.4   ANALYSING THE MARKET: WHAT PRODUCT IS NEEDED?

There are several steps when using a marketing approach to generating change. Taking aspirin as our example, the first goal was to find out what our 'customers' thought about systematically prescribing it for secondary prevention, what barriers and obstacles they perceived and what they felt they stood to gain from involvement in the FACTS Aspirin Programme. In short we had to *analyse the market*. To do this, we held a series of semi-structured interviews with general practitioners, consultants and public health consultants, continuing until no new information was being generated. In our experience this takes somewhere from 6–12 interviews.

This process defines the obstacles as perceived by potential customers and will reveal many of their motivations and inhibitions regarding the change.

10.5   DEVELOPING THE PRODUCT

With this knowledge, it is possible to devise a set of strategies and aids to overcome the obstacles. In marketing terms this *product development* ensures that what is offered will be perceived by the practitioner as helping him or her and hence is likely to be well received. In the case of the Aspirin Programme the main barrier reported by general practitioners was 'too much work, not enough time'. In response to this, we devised an Aspirin Pack styled on pharmaceutical company material, which aimed to do as much of the work as possible for participants (see Box 10.1). The pack included a summary of the evidence, a step-by-step guide to implementing the programme in the practice, leaflets for patients, postgraduate education allowance financial options, and administrative aids such as stickers for notes.

10.6   GETTING TO MEET THE CUSTOMER

The next step is to secure an initial expression of interest, a foot in the door. Initially, we mimicked the pharmaceutical industry by erecting drug stands at

---

Box 10.1   Range of materials included in the Aspirin Pack

- Promotional materials to recruit practices and to prompt clinicians to carry out the change.
- A pre-prepared audit programme.
- Practice-based, PGEA approved, training programmes.
- Synthesized evidence.
- Endorsement by local pharmaceutical and cardiology consultants.
- Administrative aids for the practices such as note identifiers and stickers.
- Individualized advice and guidance about how to implement the programme.
- Patient leaflets and letters to explain the treatment.

continuing medical education meetings to promote the programme. Later we used whatever opportunity presented itself to publicize the programme: articles in local newsletters together with brief presentations to the practice managers' forum, the fund holders' consortium, the Overseas Doctor Association, etc. Once a general practitioner had expressed interest in the programme, they were contacted by our practice worker, who deliberately cast his role as being somewhat akin to that of a pharmaceutical company representative. Gaining contact with a practice involves both persistence and a style which explicitly minimizes the disruption the contact might cause to practice routine. By this point, the marketing has metamorphosed into the next stage: the selling strategy. Once interest in the 'product' has been expressed and the representative has a foot in the door, the process of understanding the wants and needs of the customer is refined. In this way, differences between general practitioners can be discerned and accommodated.

10.7 MAKING THE CUSTOMER AWARE OF HOW YOUR PRODUCT MEETS HIS OR HER NEED

The next marketing task is to attract the *customer's attention to the lack, the hole in the market that the product is about to fill*. But simply calling attention to a lack runs the danger of inducing guilt or defensiveness. Ultimate participation is more likely if:

- The customer also has help meeting this obligation.
- And at the end of the process feels good about what they have committed themselves to doing rather than feeling policed or guilty at not having done it before.

Most practices were aware that aspirin was indicated for secondary prevention. So, the 'hole' that we aimed to fill was neither the drug itself, nor the indications for its use. Instead, researching the market had informed us that what practices wanted was simple, dependable help with the work load of actually getting aspirin to patients. One solution to this problem would have been either to have paid practices to do the work, another to have done the work for them, but lack of resources made both approaches impractical. It was therefore essential that our 'product' (the Aspirin Programme) did indeed do its job well: practices had to be able to see that by joining in the programme their work would be kept to an absolute minimum. Many practices were receptive to this approach because they perceived the use of aspirin in secondary prevention to be part of their core professional task. Participating in the programme activity helped them to be better professionals. In addition, it came from a supportive general practice organization with no performance management or policing agenda.

At this point, some practices voiced an unexpected problem – they thought they had already 'done' aspirin and that all their at risk patients had already been considered. Here we needed a strategy which could check the truth of this claim (it being notoriously easy to think that one has done something when one has not) without offending anyone. Fortunately, we had already conceived of the Aspirin Programme as a way for general practitioners city-wide to demonstrate the excellence of their service. We were thus able to say, 'Well it's great that you've done this already. Could we just have your figures to add to everyone else's? We can then demonstrate that general practitioners have "got their house in order".'

All practices approached in this way happily re-ran the relevant searches. In all but two cases (both of whom had previously applied for specific money to review their prescribing of aspirin), the computer runs showed that the practice had around the same percentage of its high risk patients on aspirin as everyone else (i.e. 45–50%), and all subsequently joined the programme.

10.8   PREPARATION

Before initiating a first visit to a practice, drug representatives learn about their product so they will be able to discuss its pros and cons to the satisfaction of the customer. They then put a lot of effort into finding out about the practice. They ask other representatives what they know about it or local pharmacists – if they are on good terms. They read the firm's records of visits made by preceding representatives. Is it an academic practice – one that might be keen to audit their work and demonstrate success? Or one primarily motivated by money? Do they want to expand their list size, so might they be interested in developing new services? Do the general practitioners have a commitment to an extended primary health care team or do they prefer to be a small single-handed practice? In which case, what style of service are they likely to be committed to? Are they fund-holders? If so, which of the incentives is likely to be in the forefront of their mind? If they are non-fund holders, how might the local hospital and health authority policies affect them? What are the special clinical interests of the partners?

On arrival at the practice, the drug representatives will carry out a rapid appraisal. What clinics do they advertise in the waiting room? If they advertise a well woman clinic, they will probably be interested in osteoporosis. If they advertise a well man clinic they may well be interested in benign prostatic hypertrophy. The size and presentation of the practice will also give an indication of its organizational capacity. It may be possible to discern whether or not it is an open organization or rigid and closed. Do the practice staff appear overworked but happy, or overworked and depressed?

10.9   THE INTERVIEW

Once successfully through the door of the consulting room, time is of the essence. Whilst representatives aim to have an enormous amount of information in their head, they only expect to draw on a tiny proportion of it. Their aim is to build on the existing enthusiasms, interests and motivations of the customer. The preparation should have helped them to identify some of these. The first few minutes of conversation after introduction will continue to build the picture which then needs to be constantly reviewed and reassessed. They may have very clear views on a subject in which case the representative may need to challenge their view and open their mind to consider alternatives. On the other hand, they may feel very uncertain and need whatever back up necessary to bolster their confidence.

10.10   GAINING CREDIBILITY

The representative then *responds* to the customer. Unlike the academic world where people are likely to want to prove they know a lot about a given subject to give them credibility, the commercial world has a different and somewhat pragmatic approach. They want to demonstrate that their product meets the needs of the customer, that it will make life easier for them. Only the information that will encourage or interest the customer is necessary. This may vary widely, depending on the individual general practitioner and their attitude toward drug representatives or whoever is in front of them. Some general practitioners view drug representatives as an opportunity for light relief from their very demanding job. Others may value the opportunity to be kept up to date on the latest research, albeit a somewhat partial account. Some may be interested in free gifts. Others may welcome an audit design that can be implemented simply and does not require any extra thought.

The representative aims to be viewed in a positive light; they want their customer to trust them, to perceive them as there to help, someone who will remove difficulties. In this way, they establish their credibility with the general practitioner. In short, they aim to be part of the 'solution', never part of the 'problem', to show interest in the customer and to have plenty of action plans (Harping and Walton, 1987). If a practice wished to adapt the programme in new and unexpected ways, this was not viewed by us a problem as it might have been had FACTS been an orthodox research programme. Instead, we tried to encourage such innovation and to learn from it ourselves.

10.11   COMMITMENT: ASKING FOR THE BUSINESS

Finally, of course, it is necessary for practices to actually commit themselves to participate. In sales speak this is known as 'Asking for the business'. Initially, we felt rather hesitant about doing this – we might precipitate rejection or place the doctor in a difficult position. In fact, getting people to commit themselves is an essential part of any change process and we soon became more adept and comfortable at it. Judging the right point to ask 'Are you going to do the Aspirin Programme then?' and doing it in such a way that people feel good about being asked is a key part of effective selling.

10.12   FOLLOW-UP

Having got to the point where the customer commits him/herself, two further steps are important:

- Arrange some sort of follow-up.
- Leave!

Follow-up is clearly important. Having committed themselves, general practitioners knew they were not alone; someone, the FACTS practice worker, was around to help should unanticipated problems develop. From our point of view, it was also important to be able to check out how the work was progressing. Some brief arrangement to telephone in a week or so and see how things are, together with ensuring that contact numbers are easily available, is all that is needed.

Leaving is perhaps an odd point to make. In selling terms, however, it is all too easy to labour a particular feature, or prolong discussing a potential problem. Both of these run the risk of wasting time and may cause the customer to review their decision. Hence it really is important to know when to leave.

Whilst drawing heavily on the techniques adopted by drug representatives, our practice worker found that being perceived as a drug representative could sometimes be a disadvantage. On occasion, it became important for him to disassociate himself from a variety of other organizations. He found it useful to be able to say, quite categorically, that he was simply there to help the practice, he did not have any other underlying motives such as profit or performance management, and this undoubtedly contributed to the programme's success. A marketing and selling strategy for this kind of programme therefore covers these main points:

1. Analyse the market: ask people what the barriers, obstacles and motivations are in the area you want to change.

2. Develop the product: knowing the obstacles, you can devise ways to over-come them, providing a variety of 'hooks' to appeal to different interests and enthusiasms.
3. Reaching the customer: getting in the door.
4. Gaining credibility: responding to the customer.
5. Getting commitment: asking for the business.
6. Follow-up.

10.13 CONCLUSION

Successfully helping change to emerge is not a right or a function commendable by virtue of one's status – it has to be earned. To be effective, those aiming to create change need both trust and credibility with as many players as possible. Honesty and a degree of independence from any single major interest group are essential. Change takes time to take root and become established. The local conditions are important – what works in one place may not work in another, and analysing and preparing the soil is at least as important as disseminating the seed. Local obstacles may need to be overcome or local variants developed.

The academic world prides itself on the completeness of its theoretical under-standing. When discussing their findings academics expect to be challenged and to be able to refute all comers. At times, being adversarial and impenetrable seem almost to be regarded as virtues. By contrast, the marketing world prides itself on the ease with which ideas can be grasped and the client's needs met. Marketing techniques have much to offer when translating research findings into action. The danger of this approach is that it can appear to be manipulative or only concerned in promoting a product. Clinicians know all too well that this is often what pharmaceutical companies are really interested in. We believe that change agents within the NHS are, in some ways, better placed to use market-ing techniques than the commercial world itself since they are free of the taint of promoting for profit. Marketing approaches are most likely to be successful when they are:

- Credible – evidence-based, practical and useful.
- Based on careful market research to identify and solve obstacles.
- Followed through with selling techniques, the essence of which is develop-ing trust and credibility with the customer and knowing when and how to press for a decision.
- Seen as part of a repertoire of ways to help people change.

The NHS has tended to have a rather narrow approach to changing clinical behaviour. Not only has the language embodied a rather limited set of assump-tions, but we have also chosen from a rather limited range of interventions. As confidence grows, then hopefully knowledge and skills from other fields, including marketing and selling, will be used with increasing confidence and effectiveness.

10.14   SUMMARY POINTS

- Existing ways of thinking, evident in metaphors, can limit the ability to implement change in health care.
- Marketing has a different approach, and a different set of metaphors, and when used appropriately has much to offer when implementing the findings of research.
- Practical techniques can be acquired by many staff who lead audit or implementation of research.
- Marketing is most likely to be successful if the techniques are credible, based on market research, followed through with selling techniques, and when seen as one part of a repertoire of implementation methods.

REFERENCES

Black N and Mays N (1996) What is 'development'? *J Health Serv Research Policy* **1**:183–184.

Dawson S (1995) Never mind the solutions: what about the issues? Lessons of industrial technology transfer for quality of health care. *Quality in Health Care* **4**:197–201.

Dennett D (1993) *Consciousness Explained*. Harmondsworth: Penguin Books, p. 301.

Dickinson E (1995) Using marketing principles for health care development. *Quality in Health Care* **4**:40–44.

Grol R (1997) Beliefs and evidence in changing clinical practice. *BMJ* **315**:418–421.

Harping G and Walton P (1987) *Bluff Your Way in Marketing*. Horsham: Ravette Books Limited.

Hodgkin P (1985) Medicine is war and other medical metaphors. *BMJ* **291**:181–182.

Lakoff G and Johnson M (1980) *Metaphors We Live By*. Chicago: Chicago University Press.

Morone JA (1986) Seven laws of policy analysis. *Journal of Policy Analysis and Management* **5**:817–819.

Soumerai S and Avorn J (1990) Principles of educational outreach (academic detailing) to improve clinical decision making. *JAMA* **263**:549–554.

INDEX

Note: Page references in *italics* refer to Figures; those in **bold** refer to Tables

accident and emergency medicine, case
    study   58–66
accountability   153
action   53–4
activists   79
Agency for Health Care Policy and
    Research (AHCPR)   28
Aspirin Programme   172–4
assessment
    audit as form of   69–72
    of options for change   74
    weaknesses   70
audit
    initiation   102, 106
    models   8
    projects   22
    protocols   28
    reports   **23**, 74
        findings   **24**
    research   162
    training   91
    see also clinical audit; interface audits
audit cycle   72–4, *73*
    and learning process   84–8, *84, 87*
    steps completed   **105**
    steps involved   104

backshooting   128
back stabbing   128
BARRIERS instrument   62
behaviour change   38, 41
behaviourism   74
behaviouristic principles   76–7
blockages   151
bottlenecks   151
breast examinations   31
bullying   128

cause and effect diagram   *6*
change
    assessment of options for   74
    facilitation frameworks   40–50
    forces promoting   39
    forces resisting   39
    and innovation   147–8
    justification   21
    obstacles, *see* obstacles to change
    potential obstacles   41
    pressures for and against   41
    reducing resistance   86
    resistance to   149
    as response to pressures   39
    strategies   **46–8, 54**
    theory   **46–8**
    see also organizational change
change agents   38
change implementation   4–7
    case study   58–66
    interface audit   96
    management role in   133–43
    method   7
    overcoming obstacles   57–67
    practical issues   5
    scenario one   65
    scenario two   66
    timetable   7
    traditional method   57–9
change management
    brief history   37–8
    and internal communications
        145–66
    systematic approach   37–57
channelling   128
childhood accidental injury
    information   32

clinical audit
  brief description   2–8
  definition   1–2
  early developments   135–7
  as form of assessment   69–72
  future relationship with
      management   140–2
  introduction   137–40
  judgement and development in   70
  and learning process   69–94
  primary purpose   70
  role in changing performance   1–19
  selection of topic   3
  shared approach   135–42
  specific characteristics   72
  specification of desired
      performance   3–4
clinical practice guidelines   27
clinical records   33
Cochrane collaboration review   11
Cochrane Effective Practice and
      Organisation of Care Review
      Group   9
cognitive learning   75
Commission for Health Improvement
      (CHI)   142
commitment   124, 176
communication   127
  culture   163
  current practice   162
  implications   145–66
  and innovation   148–50
  and organizational success   146–7
  sources   163
  staff satisfaction   162
  standards   162
  strategy   161–3
  targets   162
  upwards   159
  see also internal communication
communication audit   152–4
  comparisons with other audits   154
  definition   153
  measures employed   154–7
  outcomes   157–61
communication channels   126, 158, 159
communication drivers   158
communication review   161
communication skills training (CST)   161
communication team   159
constructivism   76
contemplators   53
continuing education   83

continuing professional development   83
continuous quality improvement
      (CQI)   14
corporate identity vs. geographic
      location   160
credibility   175
criteria   3–4, 22–4, 76
  compliance with   26
  criticisms   26
  diabetes care   4
  evidence-based   26–8
  explicit   25, 76
  implicit   25
critical reflection   79
cross-functional organizational
      teams   146
culture   45
current performance, data collection   29
customer interaction   172–4

data analysis   4, 29, 34, 103
data collection   103, 125–6
  current performance   29
  first   4, 59
  rules   29
  second   8, 30, 32, 60
data extraction   29, 33–4
decision-making   149, 159, 162
delays before emergency surgery   32
delegation of operational tasks   147
descriptive reflection   79
descriptive writing   79
development   71
  language   169
diabetes care, criterion   4
diary analysis   157
disillusion with audit   24
dissemination, language   169–70
dominance   128–9
dysfunctional teams   49

education
  and audit   82–3
  materials   9
  medical   83
  outreach   10
  programmes   38
  strategies   9–12
  see also training
emergency surgery, delays before   32
emotional reaction   45
emotions   168
empowerment   163

epidemiological studies   24
evaluations   23
evidence   21–36
    about appropriate care   24–6
    current performance   29–34
evidence-based criteria   26–8
    development methods   27–8
evidence-based standards   86
Evolution of Clinical Audit, The   82
experiential learning   75
explicit criteria   25, 76
external communication   153

fact finding   73
fairness   71
Family Health Services Authorities   137
Family Practitioner Committees   137
fear   124–5
    reducing   125–7
feasibility   71
feedback   9
fishbone diagrams   5
'five whys' approach   5
focus groups   156
follow-up   176–7
Framework for Appropriate Care
        Throughout Sheffield
        (FACTS)   167, 172

gatekeeping   128
general practitioners   40, 137
geographic location vs. corporate
        identity   160
grapevine   158
grooming behaviour   129
group audit work   85
group behaviour   44, 96
group composition   99, 103, 106–7
group experiences   109–12
group functioning   96
group level   **47**
group size   96, 99, 106–7
group task   96
group work   96, **106**
    case study   108–12
    see also interface audits; teamwork
groupthink   44, 49
growth theories   81

hormone replacement therapy   31
hypotheses
    defining   51
    generation   50–1, **52**

implementation, language   170
implementation strategies   8–17
    applications   **16**
    combinations   14–15
    selection   42, 50, 63–6
implementing change, *see* change
        implementation
implicit criteria   25
individual behaviour   43
individual obstacles and theories   45
informality promotion   163
information
    accumulation   153
    dissemination   125–6
    lack of   157–8
    timeliness   158–9
innovation
    and change   147–8
    and communication   148–50
    main features   147
    successful adoption   152
innovation curve   40–1, *41*
innovativeness, and internal
        communication   151–2
interactive episodes, self-reports of   157
interface audits   95–117
    areas covered   **103**
    case study   109–12
    change implementation   96
    experiences   104, **106**
    factors facilitating future   **108**
    factors influencing views   105–16
    future activities   108
    implications for implementing change
        in   112–16
    lessons learnt for future   107–8
    national survey   98, 102
    representation of health care
        professions   **104**
    respondents positively endorsing
        statements about experiences   **107**
    subjective experiences   98
    see also group work
internal communication
    and change management   145–66
    and innovativeness   151–2
    positive benefits   146
    and receptivity to change   151
interpersonal encounters,
        recordings   156–7
interpersonal relationships   152
interviews   63, **64**, 156, 175
involvement   124

job satisfaction   152
judgement   *71*

knowledge seeking   77, 78

language   168–71
  development   169
  dissemination   169–70
  implementation   170
  research   169
leadership   130, 141
learning cycle   *80*
learning orientations   77
learning process
  approaches   **83**
  and audit cycle   84–8, *84*, *87*
  for audit skills required   90–1
  based on audit   88–90
  case study   88, **89**
  and clinical audit   69–94
  definition   75
  development orientations   82
  individual nature of   76
  methodology   77–8
  perspectives   74–6
  reflection in   78–80
learning styles   79–80

management by expression   150
management by suppression   150
management role in change
        implementation   133–43
management strategies   150
management styles   150–1
management systems, creation   153
management's commitment and
        support   126
manipulation   129–30
Mann–Whitney test   32
market analysis   171–2
marketing
  approach   170–1
  techniques   171
medical audit advisory groups
        (MAAGs)   98, 103, 137
medical audit committee (MAC)   98, 103
medical education   83
meetings
  duration   99, 103, 105–6
  unproductive   161
meningitis in children   31
methodological problems   24
missing notes   *6*

models of audit   8
models of change   52–4
monitoring   24, 72, 73, 125–6
mounting behaviour   128–9
mourning loss   43
myocardial infarction   7

naive behaviourism   75
National Health Service, *see* NHS
National Institute of Clinical Excellence
        (NICE)   142
new practice, implementing   74
Newton's third law   39–40
NHS administrator   137
NHS efficiency index   137
NHS manager   137

observable behaviour   75
obstacles to change   **46–8**, 49, 124
  assessment   64
  identifying   59–63
  potentially successful strategies   64
  reviewing information   64
open management and organizational
        change   150–1
opinion leaders   11
organizational change   14
  and open management   150–1
  and relationship with immediate
        managers   150
organizational goals   147
organizational integrity   151
organizational level   **48**, 49–50
organizational loyalty   146
organizational restructuring   146
organizational structure   152
organizational theories   45

Pareto charts   5
patient mediated interventions   12
patient population   29–30
performance change   1–19
performance improvement, practical
        issues   5–7
performance indicators   76
performance requirement   3–4
personal behavioural change   163
personal growth and development   81
personal level   **46**
persuasion   74, 75
policy decisions, implications of   163
poorly (performing) doctor   170

power sources 45
pragmatists 79
precontemplation 52
preparation 53, 174
primary care 95
primary–secondary care interface 96
  audit initiation 98
  audits taking place at 99
  experiences of audits taking place
    100–1
  survey of audit activity 97–101
product development 172
product requirements 171–2
professionalism 134–5
psychological theories 42–4, 49
published audits, review 22–4

quality, definition 125
quality assurance activities 40
quality improvement 42
quality management technique 5
questionnaires 62, 155
  postal survey 97, 97

random sampling 33
re-engineering 146
reflection 73, 75
  for action 79
  in action 78
  on action 78–9
  in learning process 78–80
reflective learning 76, 79
reflectors 79
reliability 71
reminders 13
research
  guidance 61–2
  language 169

samples and sampling 29, 30–3
secondary care 95
  see also primary–secondary care
    interface
self-directed learning 78
self-efficacy 43
self-managed teams 146

self-reports of interactive episodes 157
selling techniques 171
senior management, visibility 160
senior management commitment 162
short-termism 76
social facilitation 44
social influence
  and conformity 44
  theory 43, 45
staff empowerment 147
standards 3–4, 73, 76
  communication 162
  developing 125
  evidence-based 86
student learning 75
symptoms of disease 42

task allocation 103
team briefing 163
team development 147
teamwork 119–32
  case study 131
  cross-functional 146
  obstacles from members 124
  problem behaviours 127–31
  resistance to participation 127
  stages of team growth and
    development 121–3
  strategies for achieving positive
    interdependence 121
  types of teams 120–1
  see also group work
theorists 79
thrombolytic treatment 7, 57
total quality management (TQM) 14, 152
training 91
  see also education
transition processes 53
transtheoretical model 44, 52–4
trust 124–5, 127
  and interaction 150

understanding seeking 77, 78

validity 71

Index compiled by Geoffrey Jones